4-14-92

9-12-92

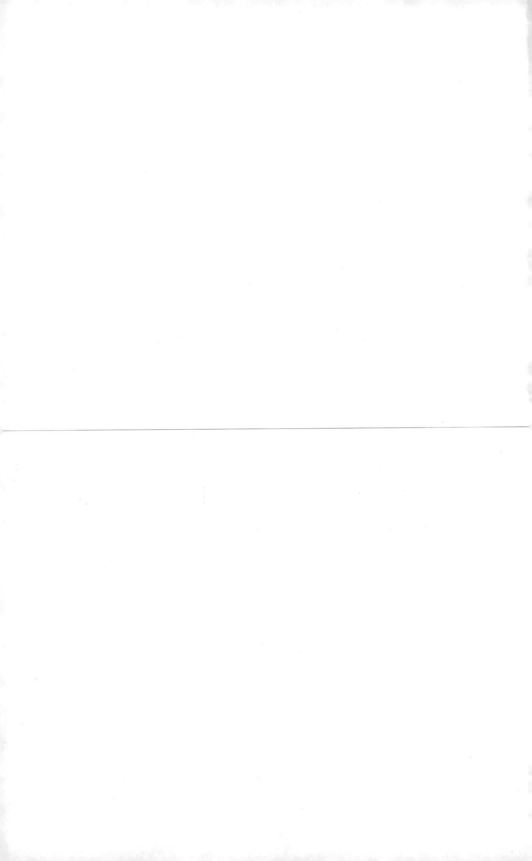

OFF
THE
PEDESTAL

TRANSFORMING THE
BUSINESS OF MEDICINE

Michael A. Greenberg, M.D.

OFF THE PEDESTAL

Published by
BREAKTHRU PUBLISHING
P.O. Box 2866
Houston, Texas 77252-2866
(713) 522-7660

Printed in the United States of America

This book is dedicated to my wife, Geri, and my daughters, Renée and Heidi, who fill my life with joy and love.

ACKNOWLEDGMENTS

I wish to acknowledge Bob and Leah Schwartz without whose vision, love, and persistence this book would have remained an unexpressed idea. Also Frank Reuter, Ph.D., my editor, who brought form from the void and made the task of writing fun. And finally, a special acknowledgment to my family, friends, teachers, colleagues, and patients who fill my life with happiness and wonderment.

INTRODUCTION

Medicine is a profession in crisis. This is, of course, no secret. On an almost daily basis, the media makes the public aware of problems in the medical profession. Malpractice premiums have become so expensive that, in some parts of the country, general practitioners no longer deliver babies; even obstetricians are giving up on their speciality. Technological advances, coupled with increases in hospital and physicians' fees, cause medical costs to greatly exceed the inflation rate. The financial effects ripple out and influence the public at large. Major corporations try to pull back from their commitment to covering health insurance costs. In an attempt to protect their benefits, workers strike as they did against several of the baby Bell telephone companies. People not covered by company health plans are threatened by the ever increasing cost of health insurance premiums, and millions have no medical coverage of any kind. In areas where poverty is prevalent, those who lack insurance are often forced to seek medical treatment at hospital emergency rooms because, by law, patients cannot be turned away. But so many patients seek care in this fashion that emergency rooms are flooded, placing great stress on hospital personnel. Not surprisingly, these critical problems influence talented young students who might make medicine a profession. Medical school applications have dropped sharply, as have the test scores of the applicants. Thus, the crisis threatens not only physicians, but society as a whole.

Is the situation hopeless? Amongst my fellow physicians, I hear much grumbling and many fatal predictions. When I tell my colleagues that the situation can be improved, most are skeptical. Threatened by the specter of socialized medicine, physicians complain vehemently but, feeling powerless, do not act. My own preference has been to attack local problems in the hopes of discovering solutions which may work on a nationwide basis. I have concluded that many of the problems which plague medicine can best be addressed by non-political solutions. If physicians and the public work together on the local level, the quality of medical care can improve, and some of the worst problems will abate.

This book, then, is an attempt to spell out the problems which trouble the medical profession and, consequently, society as a whole, and to offer recommendations about how and what can be done to alleviate the problems. The book does not merely deal with the technical or legal questions associated with health care; it is partly a tale of my own personal experiences because what happened to me is, I am quite sure, symptomatic of prevalent trends. The recommended solutions do not, for the most part, require legislation, nor are they directed only at physicians. To make medicine work, the society as a whole will have to contribute to the solutions.

A necessary first step in attempting to solve any problem is accurately defining its causes. While fully conceding that the problems of modern medicine are complex, I would contend that the causes can be understood and that the problems can be corrected through concerted physician and patient action. The following discussion will briefly identify the problems; the text will expound on them and offer solutions.

The first and greatest problem which plagues medicine is the age old problem of human greed. Our society as a whole has been overwhelmed by materialism. Amidst plenty, we all seem to want a greater and greater personal share of available resources. Although I am referring to physician greed—my own included—the issue is much larger. Medicine has become big business, and as such, those involved in it—physicians, other health care practitioners, insurance companies, special interest groups, politicians, lawyers, yes and even patients—are all partly to blame. Physicians too often set their rates as if their payments on a Mercedes are the basis for fees. Special interest groups work to reduce the health costs of those they represent, in effect, shifting the burden to other segments of the population. Lawyers accept frivolous malpractice suits in the hopes of making a big killing. Politicians make proposals based on public appeal, not on the best interests of the body politic. And insurance companies resist scrutiny regarding margins of profit. When I point the finger here, I point it first at myself. In fact, as the book will show, some of my recommendations for reform arise from my personal attempts to deal with the concept of a "fair share."

A second cause of the crisis in medicine is patient failure to take responsibility for health. Too often, patients feel as if doctors should carry the full burden of keeping them healthy, no matter how they have treated their own bodies. What I will have to say about this issue is not new; for several years the media has given much attention to issues of health—the highly organized attack on smoking being an obvious example—but more needs to be said.

The increasing dependence on technological solutions to medical problems is a third cause. Modern medicine has, to a great extent, become technologically oriented. The media reports regularly on modern medical "miracles": the replacement of the human heart with an artificial one, organ transplants, and the use of sophisticated equipment in the diagnosis of disease. Though this technology is admittedly awe inspiring, the general public hears so much about radical procedures that many people are left with the impression that medicine can and ought to do anything and everything to restore a person to "health." Often, however, these technical solutions, while being able to sustain life, cannot improve its quality. And in some cases, physicians treat the technology as if it were more important than the patients—with their hopes, fears, and concerns for well-being.

The fourth problem is the malpractice crisis. Huge monetary settlements drive up the cost of physicians' insurance. Part of these costs are passed on to patients, either directly in the form of higher fees or indirectly in increases in health insurance premiums. But the malpractice crisis has another dimension which, though less publicized, is of equal or greater importance because it directly affects patients and the quality of the treatment they receive. Any physician who practices in an emergency room will tell you that he or she must now practice as if an additional silent partner were in the room—an attorney. Virtually every patient who is treated in an emergency room and who *may* have had a head

INTRODUCTION

or internal injury will be X-rayed even when the
physician thinks the procedure is not necessary
and the patient would be better off without the
exposure to the radiation. The physician, however, must order the X-rays just in case a patient
were to sue. In fact, in all medical fields, doctors
are practicing medicine defensively in order to
protect themselves, often at the cost of giving
optimal care. Doctors are being *forced* to ask
themselves the question "What is best for the
law?" not "What is best for the patient?"

A recent event saddened me deeply. I had been
talking with a just retired doctor and had eagerly
passed on the word that the son of a common
friend had decided to enter the medical profession. The young man had been accepted into
a competitive undergraduate school, one which
has an excellent record of placing its students in
top medical universities. The doctor, a man I
respect deeply because he was a caring physician,
responded bitterly: "I wouldn't advise anyone to
go into medicine now. Even before I retired, my
hands were tied. How can anyone expect us to
practice medicine well if a government agent or
a lawyer tells us what is best for our patients?
It's just foolish."

Foolishness must stop. Read this text and do
your part.

Section I

THE SERVICE OF HUMANITY

The old ideas are new again because they are not old; they are timeless: duty, sacrifice, commitment . . .

George Bush
Inaugural Address

May the love of my art actuate me at all times; may neither avarice nor thirst for glory or ambition for reputation engage my mind, for enemies of truth and philanthropy, they could easily deceive me and make me forgetful of my lofty aim of doing good to Thy children.

Maimonides

THE SERVICE OF HUMANITY

Now being admitted to the profession of medicine, I solemnly pledge to consecrate my life to the service of humanity. . . . The life and health of my patient will be my first consideration.

The Oath of Hippocrates

2

Chapter I

A CAREER SIDETRACKED

My choice of medicine as a profession was motivated by a strong desire to help people and by a fascination with the structure of the human body. Coincidentally, I also knew that the profession would provide me with an above average income and allow me to lead a comfortable life and support a family. I see no contradiction in those goals: being an excellent physician and supporting one's family comfortably. Doctors as much as anyone else are committed to providing for the well-being of their loved ones. One does not have to follow St. Francis, giving up all worldly goods, to serve mankind. In fact, when I decided to enter medicine, I was consciously modeling my life on that of my family physician, Dr. Charles Beck, Sr.

Dr. Beck's medical ethics were above reproach. His attitude toward the practice of medicine and his handling of patients motivated at least one other young man to enter the medical profession: his own son, Chuck. During a visit to his father's office, the younger Beck once saw his father cut a patient's toenails. As soon as Charles Jr. had an opportunity to talk privately with his father, he rebuked him, contending that it was undignified for a physician to perform such a humble act. The father calmly explained to his son that caring for his patients was not in any way demeaning, but an act of love. The patient in question was poor and had physical problems which limited his dexterity. Had he developed an infection, he would not have been able to afford a podiatrist. The lesson was well learned; on a later occasion, Dr. Beck Sr. saw his son cutting the toenails of a patient.

That attitude of service made us feel as if Charles Beck was more than just our doctor; he seemed to be a part of our family. We all knew that he always had our best interests at heart. My mother, who was plagued by illnesses and needed several operations, trusted Dr. Beck's judgments implicitly and willingly placed her life in his hands. She also credited him with saving my own life at the age of ten. I never recall any discussion about Dr. Beck administering unnecessary medical treatment, and he certainly never was criticized for charging too much or making financial reward the primary focus of his life. We had complete trust in this man.

Oh, there were complaints. At times his office was busy and we had to wait a long time to see him. But, even if my mother became angry at him for the long waits, she always forgave him. She knew that when it was her turn to be seen by the doctor, he would not rush her and that the long waits were a result of the doctor's offering his patients detailed advice. Because he was devoted to our welfare, Dr. Beck held a position in our family only a step lower than an angel.

And we loved him in spite of the fact that he was a bit of an eccentric. He spent hours at the Salvation Army resale shop collecting various bits of refuse. Years later, he appeared on the Oprah Winfrey show, not because of his medical knowledge, but because of his pack-rat behavior. In a pinch, he once used half of a rubber ball as part of a bandage on my arm. He certainly was different than us in many ways: he drove a better car than we did, but that didn't seem to bother us or anyone else. He had a boat which he used for weekend recreation, but like the car, we wanted him to have that because he worked so

5

hard. When we needed him, he was always there and we knew he cared.

Dr. Beck's personal life was probably disrupted a great deal. He never did get to spend much time on his boat. Hopefully, however, his wife and children understood that he was dedicated to his practice. Time spent away from them was always devoted to helping patients. His children may have suffered from the fact that he wasn't around as much as other fathers, but that was the price to be paid by his choice in becoming a physician. On the other hand, his dedication and care offered his children a model of a life devoted to serving one's fellow man.

Doctor Beck made his choice to enter medicine freely, knowing that he would have to sacrifice to bring excellence to the profession. Medicine, at that time, was practiced by placing one's patients before one's own needs and wants. Advertising or public promotion of one's practice was strictly forbidden by the code of ethics of the American Medical Association. Doctors were not high-pressure businessmen; they permitted patients who had financial burdens to delay payment. Certainly all physicians were not Charles Becks, but in those days it seems that it was easier to find a physician more dedicated to his patients than to making large amounts of money.

Dr. Beck represents for me a lost ideal—one that needs to be re-established. My goal when I first entered the profession was to emulate Dr. Beck—to offer services as he did and to accept as my reward the appreciation and respect of my patients. Regrettably, though well motivated, I became sidetracked. My story is long and contains some digressions not directly related to medicine, but it will serve as a fairly typical example of how easily a physician can be distracted from practicing medicine as he should.

Even before I began practicing medicine, I was rudely introduced to a level of greed in the profession which disturbed me. While serving my residency, quite a few of my fellow residents began taking moonlighting jobs, mostly as part of what was called the 'earlobe empire,' piercing ears in department stores. Having come from a family of modest means—I had lost my father at an early age—and eager to begin earning money, I too began piercing ears until one of us was seen by a professor—a sighting which caused the suffering of terminal embarrassment. The medical school administration said nothing about our working outside our residency as long as what we did was legal and respectable. None of the residents, however, wanted to openly discuss moonlighting with the faculty for a rather simple reason: working weekends, we were able to earn as much as our professors were earning teaching in medical school.

Residents also had many opportunities to work in offices for dermatologists. Some of these physicians ran practices which were models of caring while others were factories in which patients were run through as though they were goods on a conveyer belt. Within the walls of a university medical center hospital, students and residents have very little idea of what the outside world of medical practice is really like. Our eyes were quickly opened; the clinics in which we worked seemed to treat a never ending stream of patients. Because, as part-time help, the residents had not created the heavy scheduling problems, we developed a rather callous attitude: move the patients through the clinic as efficiently as possible so that we would be able to get off work at a reasonable hour. After all, we had other responsibilities.

In the private offices I observed or heard about, the same attitude was present. Patients were viewed as numbers. Often they were kept waiting for extended periods before they were examined, and then insufficient time would be allotted for a complete examination of their medical problems. I promised myself that when I established my own practice, my patients would not be kept waiting, and I would not be rushed when I tended to their needs.

8

One problem I became aware of was that patients who came into some of these offices or clinics knew little about the maladies for which they were being treated. Commonly they would ask questions by stumbling over some big words which had been thrown at them during an earlier visit. The medical profession, like all technical professions, has a specialized language necessary to facilitate work. Doctors speak a particular jargon that allows them to communicate clearly among themselves. When doctors speak to patients, however, they sometimes forget that patients never learned the medical language. One of my goals was to translate to each patient the meaning of the specialized terms which might otherwise confuse them, and I resolved that when I began practicing I would speak to each patient in plain English. Patients, after all, should understand the nature of their problems and the purpose of any prescribed medication, including all common side effects or complications which might occur.

Some of my rather rude experiences in residency caused me to reflect on my future and on the values which had brought me to the doorway of a new career. Determined not to repeat the mistakes of others, I developed three basic rules of medical practice for myself. By following these rules, I avoided, for a number of years, most of the standard problems which occur in my profession. I created a happy, successful practice. My rules were:

1. All patients shall be treated with as much care as if they were members of my immediate family.

2. If another physician can perform a procedure better than I can, the patient shall be referred to that doctor.

3. Always tell the truth.

The reader can see the influence of Doctor Charles Beck, Sr. in rule number one. The second and third rules made simple common sense. Armed with this philosophy and having left my need for moonlighting behind me, I had a promising career in front of me. And I received a wonderful first break. A dermatologist, Dr. John Cox, invited me to begin practicing in Elk Grove Village, Illinois. His own excellent professional reputation had led him to be vastly overbooked. Patients often had to wait four to six weeks for an appointment.

Being a decent man and a concerned doctor, John was troubled with the length of time it took for his patients to see him. He suggested that if I opened an office in the area, patients could be seen more readily. In that way, the local population would be served, he would not feel as much pressure from patients needing immediate attention, and I could build a practice quickly. The arrangement was one of those happy situations in which everyone wins. He knew he was capable of seeing only a limited number of patients every day. To see more than a specific number was to give inadequate time to *all* of his patients. That was a lesson I had already learned while moonlighting, but was eventually to forget.

John has always been concerned about and has upheld the highest standards in our specialty. His request that I accept his excess patients was a great compliment. He placed his trust in me because he felt I would practice only excellent dermatology, and he expressed delight when I agreed to open an office about fifteen minutes away from his. Because he was so busy, he was not threatened by another doctor moving so close to him.

Circumstances, however, were to change the way I practiced medicine. The changes were gradual and subtle, but they were the natural outcome of my very human instincts and needs. One by one, my ideals became threatened— without me even realizing that I was abandoning my principles.

My initial gratitude for my opportunity took a long time to erode, but the circumstances under which I worked made the change almost inevitable. Because the hospital at which I began practicing, the Alexian Brothers Medical Center, did not have a dermatologist on campus, they were so pleased to have me working with them that they let me open my office in their attached physicians' building. Offices in this building were usually reserved for doctors who admitted a large number of patients or who had patients so ill that the physicians needed to be near the hospital floors. Even though I did not fit into either category, I was given office space. In turn, I was expected to see inpatient consultations with great expediency. This arrangement satisfied me because I had already committed myself to the concept of offering prompt service.

But I quickly came to realize that many of the consultations were unnecessary. Patients who have nothing to do with their time in a hospital will often request or even demand multiple consultations. If they are troubled by minor medical problems, they feel that they might as well have everything "fixed up" during the hospital stay. Primary care doctors will often assent to their patients' requests and order the consultations, especially if they fear that patients whose demands are not satisfied might switch to another doctor. A great deal of my time in the hospital was spent seeing common skin problems which patients had tolerated for years without treatment. But I was afraid to express my feelings to my colleagues regarding the non-necessity of some of their consultations for fear they would stop sending patients to my office.

Of course, the patients were not always totally innocent. Patients understandably try to pass their medical fees on to insurance companies. Trying to take advantage of a situation is, after all, a distinctly human trait. Most of these patients knew that they should have pursued non-essential problems as outpatients either before they were admitted to, or after they were released from the hospital. They also knew that if they had sought treatment, they would have had to make a potentially inconvenient office appointment and pay for the service. It is almost as though they said, "Well, as long as I am here, I'll let my insurance pay for the problem instead of paying for it myself." Of course, the insurance companies were smart enough to know that a wart removal was not a necessary part of follow-up treatment to gall bladder surgery. The insurance companies rightfully refused payment, and I was often stuck with useless bills, which patients steadfastly refused to pay.

In addition to the insurance problem, I was often asked to attend to the acne problems of adolescents being treated in locked psychiatric units. After being billed for the visit, parents made angry phone calls to our office. The parents had not ordered the care for their children and they refused to pay because the visit was not authorized. We had no recourse with these bills and never pursued them. Occasionally

I would be asked to see inpatients who were so out of touch with reality that they denied I had ever visited them, and they refused to pay for service actually performed. Naturally, my anger with the whole system was the result of the low level of reimbursement I was receiving for inpatient hospital consultations.

What was missing in all these cases was communication. I did not explain to patients that their insurance probably would not cover preexisting conditions during a hospitalization. A physician must take a great deal of time to explain to demanding patients that unnecessary consultations are inconsiderate to a doctor who has to go out of his way to treat a problem the patient should have handled before being admitted to a hospital. Many doctors, and I was one of them, are afraid to confront their patients with the truth. Looking good to their patients and colleagues is a stronger motivating force than offering wise counsel.

Even some of my fellow physicians did not understand my feelings about consultations. I explained to them that if a problem existed, such as a drug reaction, in which the patient was in discomfort, I would be at the hospital immediately and did not care if the patient ever paid. I also tried to convey to my colleagues that some consultations, which may technically be classified as unnecessary, make an enormous difference in a patient's life. Elderly people or those who have difficulty traveling to a physician's office should be seen in a hospital as a convenience to them. I welcomed these consultations even though, in the strictest sense, they are not necessary on an inpatient basis. The cosmetic help does make a difference in these patients' lives and I am glad to help them, even without reimbursement. But in most cases, I was being asked to work for free on problems which were not medically significant. A small number of colleagues were guilty, in my opinion, of putting their own image with their patients ahead of my need to serve my own clientele.

My businesslike attitude toward consultations caused me to gradually isolate myself from some of my colleagues. Because I was being used on some occasions, I began to become more concerned with my reimbursement than with patient well-being. I was slowly changing from a caring doctor into a businessman. I encouraged consultations to please my fellow staff members and to maintain my status. But instead of communicating my true feelings of resentment to my fellow physicians, I allowed the anger within me to fester and I began to separate myself emotionally and even physically from the medical staff and the patients. I did not realize, nor did most people around me, how much I had grown to resent what I was doing and how I carried internal feelings of self-doubt about my performance.

As these in-hospital problems developed, my outpatient practice grew rapidly. But I found that my appointment book was never totally filled, not even a week ahead, much less the four weeks of a physician like Dr. Cox. This disturbed me because I had come to believe that a full schedule was a mark of true success. I had heard that other practices were filled days or weeks in advance and wondered why my appointment book had patient spaces available, sometimes on the same day.

What eventually became apparent to me was that I had simply created an unrealistic number of spaces in my appointment book. Many of my patients seemed satisfied with the time given to them but occasionally complaints would reach me from my office manager about patients who felt that they were being rushed. I became endlessly dissatisfied because of the silly idea in my head that success in medicine is measured by the inconvenience new patients must suffer in waiting for an appointment.

And then came the final blow to all my young, idealistic goals. After approximately eight years of practice, I was stunned to find another dermatologist moving into an office building directly across the street from the hospital. His arrival eventually led me to recommit myself to my original ideals. But first, it almost destroyed me.

The news that a new doctor had moved directly across the street reached me only after his office was open and he was a member of the staff. This came to me as a shock because, as a courtesy, new physicians normally tell established physicians when they will be moving into an area. Back when I was a resident, it was general knowledge that if one asked already established dermatologists if there was room for additional specialists in their areas, the answer would universally be negative. The result was that residents stopped asking those types of questions. If they were smart, and we all were, anonymous phone calls placed to offices would give accurate information as to the fullness of the doctor's schedule. All the resident needed to ask was how soon he could schedule an appointment for a new patient and what the fees were. This strategy helped young physicians find locations where they would be most readily accepted.

Once the location of my own office was chosen, I spoke with all the local dermatologists to let them know of my intention to move into the area and to establish communication with them. Of course, I offered to cover for them and accept any emergency care patients who could not be accommodated into their busy schedules.

You can imagine my surprise then when I realized that a dermatologist had moved in across the street from me without my knowing it. But the fault was mine, not his. Never having been one for excellent attendance at meetings, including those of my own medical department, I had never even seen his application to the staff even though applications for new staff members were available for examination at department meetings. I had no idea a new dermatologist was even considering practicing in our area. Thus, though I was at fault, I felt offended that the new doctor had not come to introduce himself to me.

What initially bothered me about a new physician opening so close to my office was the loss of my monopoly. I was the only dermatologist physically located so close to the hospital and, therefore, I received and took care of virtually all of the in-hospital consultations. Nevertheless, a dermatologist's main source of income comes from office work. Since I am a normal human being, I jealously set out to guard my territory. Another physician so close to the hospital was a threat because he also would be available for inpatient consultations. I believed that he would be able to please the physicians in the hospital by his availability and would take part of my practice away from me. I found myself becoming an angry man. Since I had obviously offended some of the attending doctors in the hospital by complaining of the way they used me on unnecessary inpatient consultations, the new physician loomed as an even larger threat. Frankly, I was scared. A story developed inside my head that, for years, success had been handed to me without effort, and now it was time to pay the piper.

Never having met the new kid on the block, I had no personal feelings for him, but everything he did shook me up. He appeared to be armed with professional practice building skills. I suspected, but did not know for sure, that he used a professional practice consultant. Every time I opened a newspaper or newsletter from a local organization, his advertisements jumped out at me. He appeared to have a slick plan for rapid growth.

He held an open house for his new office that, in my opinion, was more appropriate to the opening of a new grocery store than a doctor's office. If I had any reason to doubt the basis of my fears of undue competition, the grand opening scared me silly. My competitor arranged a photo opportunity, cutting a big red ribbon across the front of his office in the presence of the local mayor.

My feelings about the new dermatologist actually were reflections of feelings about myself. Because I had been fortunate during most of my life, circumstances allowed me to disguise the fact that I really had a very poor self-image. I was a master at hiding this fact from everyone in my world, especially myself. In fact, many who know me are shocked to know of the crisis I went through from the threat of competition; they contend that the ugly side of my actions did not show to the world at large. But I felt uncomfortable with other physicians, especially fellow dermatologists, because I came to believe that I was not as good as they were, in spite of all those years of successful practice and a loyal following of happy patients.

An insecure underside of my personality, one which had its basis in my own past experience, surfaced. From grammar school on, school had always come so easy to me that I could receive above average grades without effort. Achievement tests seemed even easier, and so, not being challenged, I became academically lazy. I was hurt several times: an elementary school teacher once unjustly questioned my mathematical ability and forever shook my confidence in my math prowess; I resented a particular college level biology course and luckily pulled out an acceptable grade on a final examination. Then when I decided to specialize in dermatology, I did not take enough time to study for the American Academy of Dermatology board exams; consequently, it took me three years to pass them. The combination of some belittling experiences and my own flippant attitude toward academics was to slip below the surface of my consciousness and to fester there. These experiences added credence to the idea that I was not as good as other physicians.

So the new dermatologist, quite apart from who he was or what he did, triggered a crisis in my own personality. My history of being able to learn easily led me to think of myself as something of a lazy fraud. I lost sight of the fact that I was a highly regarded physician and I began to fear that I was a terribly ordinary doctor.

Being an outstanding doctor is more than having a vast knowledge of all of the facts available in medicine. No one dermatologist can know everything there is to know about skin diseases. Besides mastering data and theory, doctors learn how to look up those rare problems which are encountered only a few times in a lifetime of practice. Medicine is just like any other job or profession. Most of what one sees or does everyday is repetitive and ordinary. The same few diseases make up the majority of one's daily routine. When the physician is confronted with something rare or strange, help can always be found, assuming that one's ego does not get in the way.

My ego, however, had become a problem for me. Hurt and unsure of myself, I saw the new dermatologist as a threat. My solution to my problem was to avoid contact with other physicians as much as possible. This was done so they would not discover the "truth" which I had come to believe about myself—that I was a mediocre doctor.

One way in which a new physician on a staff obtains patients is to be highly visible. This usually takes the form of hours spent drinking awful coffee and eating stale doughnuts in the physician's lounge. During that time, the new doctor has to suffer the embarrassment and fear of approaching staff physicians he has never met and introducing himself. After the new dermatologist joined the staff, it seemed that every time I passed the doctor's lounge, he was there promoting his new practice. He was, of course, doing the professionally astute thing. In my mind, my "I'm not good enough" conversation prevented me from socializing with the staff as much as I would have liked. I saw "my competition" increasing his practice and envisioned my practice declining because of his actions. I spent a great deal of time and mental energy imagining that he was wrong in everything he did, even though he was just doing what any new doctor would do to establish a practice. Needless to say, my dislike for him grew. In my mind, he was wrong for doing what was correct for his practice.

Refusing to sit back and watch as my patients moved across the street—an unrealistic fantasy, but a painful one—I began to spend more time with the staff and discovered that tea—I despised the coffee—was also available in the doctor's lounge. As normal humans, we very often do not have a sense of how much others approve of or like us. Even when they tell us, we have problems accepting the acknowledgment. But, slowly I began to regain a sense of the respect many staff members held for me. The only one who hadn't recognized that I was doing a good job was me.

Having mastered personal promotion in the lounge areas, I moved on to try to compete in the arena of advertising. When I first began practicing medicine, advertising was banned by the American Medical Association. A discrete boxed advertisement in the local papers was considered the limits of propriety, and then only to announce the opening of a new office. Along with other doctors, I had come to fear censure by the AMA for blatantly promoting my practice. But the challenge of competition caused me to drop all past inhibitions and to attempt to compete openly.

My experiments in competitive advertising took the form of ads placed in the same newspapers as my colleague across the street. Very few, if any, patients arrived at my office as a result of those ads. Advertising was not working to bring in patients and protect my standard of living. In retrospect, all the advertising money spent would have been better kept and put back into my practice or used to take an exciting vacation. When my first round of ads did not work, my next project to increase office revenue was a campaign to promote collagen injections for wrinkles. I specifically targeted the male population, which was a fresh, virtually untapped market. Older executives in competition with younger colleagues could be made to look better, thereby increasing their sense of worth. A significant amount of money was spent on a public relations representative who provided exposure on radio and television and produced a brochure for direct mail advertising to executives.

The experiment was a total failure and a waste of money. The response from the promotion did not even recover the cost of the advertising. As a physician I should have stuck to medicine; Madison Avenue was just not my calling. Had I recognized where my strengths lay, several thousand dollars would have been saved.

Certain types of promotion by the medical profession are worthwhile. These involve benefits to society in general and not to one's own pocketbook. The only positive incident which stemmed from my use of the public relations person was that I was able to help educate the public—via a brush with British royalty.

Dermatologists are strong advocates of avoiding needless exposure to the sun and are sworn enemies of artificial tanning parlors. *People* magazine reported that the Duchess of York, preparing for a visit to California, had been spending time in an English tanning parlor developing her suntan. I wrote to "Fergie" and faxed the letter to her via the British Consul in Los Angeles. The letter chastised her for her behavior. Fergie and her sister-in-law, Diana, set an example for millions of women the world over, and as a public figure, she has a responsibility to act with good judgment, or at least keep harmful practices private. A terse, typically British note was sent in response. The note stated that the Duchess had received my letter and had noted the content.

Through the effort of my publicist, the story was picked up by television, radio, and the newspapers on a national level. This publicity had a point to it: a concern for public health. My intention in sending out this message was not to promote my own practice.

The only type of publicity that worked for me was that which was not intended to increase the amount of my personal office income, but which would make a positive impact on the lives of others. Nobody seemed to be interested in me when the purpose of a news story had hidden within it my desire to make more money. I freely admit that my motive for the collagen promotion was to increase my income. Nobody was fooled into thinking I was trying to improve the lot of mankind. My little internal voice kept telling me to stop wasting time and money on personal promotion.

During this period, I also took a number of speaking engagements in the community with skin cancer prevention as the subject. The talks gave me a feeling of satisfaction. And I took part in a program sponsored by the American Academy of Dermatology, a free skin cancer screening, which has now become an annual event at our hospital. The first year, our volunteer physicians saw and screened over four hundred people from the local community. We found three melanomas that day. Melanoma is a particular type of skin cancer that spreads easily and, due to a lack of early detection, is responsible for thousands of unnecessary deaths each year. The screening was probably responsible for saving three lives. We also found a large number of abnormal moles and basal cell cancers. Basal cell skin cancers do local damage and must be removed. They generally do not spread to the rest of the body but early detection can save a patient a potentially disfiguring surgical scar.

Though these experiences gave me gratification, I was still worried about my work load.
Having realized that my advertising promotions
would not expand my business, I became determined to see that none of my patients would go
to see 'the new kid on the block' because my
schedule was too full to see them immediately.
My office staff received instructions to increase
the number of patients I saw each day, especially
during the two nights a week I stayed open until
8:30, the most popular and busy times in my
schedule because patients could see me without
losing time away from their jobs.

In an effort to please all my patients so they
would not leave me and go elsewhere—especially to the new guy across the street—my office
became just the factory type of practice I
despised during my residency. Fatigue and ir-
ritability became my constant companions. My
practice had always been fun and rewarding.
Going to my office each day had once been a joy,
not a job to be dreaded. But everything changed
in response to the threat of competition. A number of patients left my practice during that
period—not because a better doctor was practicing across the street, but because I had become a
less caring and sensitive one. I simply squeezed
too many visits into my schedule. Visits were
tense for both the patient and myself. Patients
cannot be fooled. They sense when their doctor

is concentrating more on his watch than on their care.

Any patient who demanded a larger amount of time than the minimum became a problem. If a patient had an unusual request or needed extra time to talk, I treated the patient as a nuisance for throwing my office schedule out of line. My irritation with patients was obvious, and some were correct to seek other physicians. Of course, I never saw myself as the cause of the problems. It is not human nature to place blame on oneself.

Sometimes enlightenment creeps into one's life inadvertently, like the gentle rays of the morning sun peering over the horizon. Not so for me. I slammed into a brick wall of enlightenment at about 200 miles an hour. My reawakening took place at a weekend workshop where I was forced to confront the problems which were plaguing me: my insecurity, my defensiveness, and the distortion which had taken place in my values.

Having been overweight for years—the word "husky" was to me a despised euphemism—I attended a weight-loss workshop run by Bob Schwartz, the author of **Diets Don't Work**. The workshop, to my surprise, not only dealt with practical advice about weight control; more so, it challenged participants to understand themselves and their motivations for eating too much. By the end of the weekend, I developed life changing insights, including ideas regarding my eating habits. I saw, for the first time, that I was habitually using food as a reward, as a substitute for other pleasures. I had been living by a formula which could be represented:

food = pleasure = love = comfort

All humans seek love and comfort, but when we substitute food for these essential human needs, the result is inevitable: we become fat. Once we are overweight and despise the condition, we continue to eat, either out of self-pity or as a form of self-punishment, thereby making ourselves fatter and more unhappy. I saw that I was using food to control my emotional, not my nutritional needs. I gained another important insight: this pattern had begun when I was young as an attempt to please my mother.

In spite of the fact that my mother was a loving person who was committed to my welfare, life with her was a power struggle. She was filled with anger from own her childhood and often became excessively upset with my sister and me. Like all children, I wanted to please my mother. The easiest way to achieve that goal, my mother being Jewish, was to eat excessively. DIETS DON'T WORK helped me to realize that I had developed bad habits: I used food to reduce tension and win my mother's affection.

This surprising insight led me to look carefully at other aspects of my life. When I was young, for example, I often had intense headaches which quite commonly coincided with periods during which my behavior was being questioned. But if I experienced a headache, my mother, rather than becoming angry with me, would show sympathy and gentle love. Doctors could find nothing wrong with me, and the headaches always disappeared in due time. I assume now that these headaches were created by me, without my conscious knowledge, because they served a purpose, that of reducing my mother's anger and eliciting pity.

Learning to understand my own problems and fears also helped me to understand similar problems in my patients. I once treated a woman who constantly asked me about her children's skin problems. She wanted me to diagnose her children without seeing them, even though I carefully explained to her that dermatology is a visual specialty. Aware that the cost of a visit was not the problem, I asked her about her own past experiences with doctors. In response, she spilled out her story. As a child she had multiple non-specific medical complaints for which she was taken to a doctor by her mother. The doctor, frustrated with not being able to find a cause for the complaints, humiliated her mother for continually making appointments for no apparent reason. These past episodes so controlled her present that she was afraid to bring her children to a doctor, fearing that she too would be humiliated.

In the months following the workshop, I changed my habits and gained control of my weight problem. Other seminars provided more insight into my behavior. I also began to re-evaluate the way I was practicing medicine. It became apparent that my anger and defensiveness had grown out of unjustified fears and an attempt to protect myself. I could see that my actions—my advertising campaigns, my petty anger at my colleague, and my increasingly insensitive treatment of my patients—were the grown-up's equivalent of my childhood headaches and overeating. As I came to understand some of the formative influences of my behavior, I was able to deal more openly and honestly with myself and others. I realized that I had been trying to justify the correctness of all my actions while, conversely, blaming all my problems on someone else. Luckily, all that changed. Since I no longer cultivated a great deal of internal anger, I learned to handle difficult situations with ease. Grace under pressure was mine at last.

Something, however, was still missing from my life. Then one day while waiting for a staff meeting to start, I began talking with a physician, Dr. Suhail Ghattas, to whom I had rarely spoken in the eleven years we were on the same staff.

31

Out of nowhere an intense discussion material-
ized. A veil was lifted from my face as Suhail led
me to see that my dissatisfaction with my practice was the result of my having lost sight of the
reasons why I entered medicine. In a word, I had
forgotten what I had learned from Dr. Charles
Beck about humility. I had been so threatened
by what I perceived to be a potential loss to my
income and so concerned with my professional
survival that I had been concentrating on the
business of medicine and not on the caring or
practicing side. That discussion was the starting
point of my commitment to seeing that quality
medicine would be practiced everywhere. But I
knew that I would have to begin reforming my
own habits first.

Examining my practice, I came to realize that
the first issue to be handled was the number of
patients I was seeing. Ironically, Doctor John
Cox, who helped to get me started in dermatology, dropped by for a visit just about the time I
was contemplating this question. For eleven
years my idea of success was to have an appointment book as full as his, crowded with patients
weeks in advance. Imagine my surprise and
chagrin when John told me he was actually
seeing twenty to thirty patients per day *less* than
I was. Very politely, he informed me that I was
seeing far too many patients to be giving adequate time to their needs. He was, of course,

absolutely correct, and I altered my schedule accordingly.

The next issue to be addressed was access to care for those who could not afford my services. The true joy of life comes not from fulfilling our personal needs and wants, but from stepping outside our individual needs to make a difference in the lives of other people. It became clear to me, however, that I could not, nor should not, give away more than my fair share of time to the needy. I had already experienced an erosion of my values because I had once felt "used" and tricked into doing too much work with little or no compensation.

My decision was to give away 10 percent of my practice to those who could not afford my care, an amount I considered proper for me. It is, of course, also the proportion mentioned since biblical times as a tithe. With the support of administration of the Alexian Brothers Medical Center, I opened a public aid clinic for dermatology patients. I also examined my private practice to determine where I could be of assistance to patients, especially those who might face financial difficulties. I made a promise to my patients that if they got into financial trouble, they would not be turned away from my office for lack of money.

When my patients found out what I was up to, most of them were delighted and supportive. A few had concerns about what I was doing; they were afraid I would leave private practice to work in free clinics. That fear was a great compliment from them. They were acknowledging, by expressing their fears, how much they respected me and wanted me to be their physician. Other patients were understandably concerned that I would raise my fees in order to compensate for lost income. If that were to happen, I would be taking the credit for serving non-paying patients while they would bear the cost. I assured them that although my fees might rise with time in normal fashion, I would not raise them to cover the cost of my charity work.

Once I had my own practice in order, I contemplated the next step, reaching out and working to improve medicine everywhere. The outgrowth of this concern has been the establishment of *Making Medicine Work*, a not-for-profit corporation, which is dedicated to the following promise:

By the year 2000, everyone on this planet will have access to quality health care without regard to ability to pay for the care, at the same time that physicians can support their families in comfort.

This is the promise to which I have dedicated my life. It is the fulfillment of the lesson I learned from Dr. Charles Beck.

Chapter II

REFORM

When I entered medicine, I knew that if I followed my own rules, my practice would provide excellent care for my patients and a comfortable living for my wife and children. My initial motivations were, I believe, beyond reproach. Sadly, I became sidetracked. Being all too human, I found myself threatened by competition; consequently, the quality of the services I was offering diminished. In a word, I put worries about my income ahead of concerns for my patients. What happened to me, I think, can happen to any physician—not necessarily in the same way. I responded to what I perceived was an external threat; other physicians may find themselves economically swept up by the need to maintain status via the owning of an expensive home and automobile. Whatever the reasons, I truly believe that greed or the need to protect one's own turf is at least part of the cause of our present medical crisis. My personal feeling is that the overwhelming number of my colleagues are not overly selfish or self-serving, but circumstances can lead well-meaning individuals, especially those who feel threatened, to act in greedy fashion.

The problem does not start with medicine; our society measures success in terms of the size of one's salary, the cost of one's personal possessions, and the number of connections one has in the community. Many of us act as though it were a mathematical truth that:

money = possessions = power = happiness

Money and possessions, however, do not necessarily produce happiness. Ironically, in many cases, very wealthy people are eternally dissatisfied. Once an individual obtains those possessions which were supposed to produce happiness, the person realizes that what is owned was not really what was wanted in the first place, or at least is not nearly enough. In the never ending pursuit of possessions, we tend to forget that happiness comes from self-respect and honest relationships with other people. Regrettably, our society supports the money =

36

happiness formula on a day to day basis and did so even before we existed. We had no choice but to be born into such a value system. We do, however, have the ability to alter it.

Since the great depression, the middle class in America has become increasingly wealthy and comfortable. The easy flow of goods has given rise to a consumption-oriented, status-conscious materialism. Where once families learned to repair clothes or shoes, or to make an automobile last for years, we now not only toss out good clothes just because they go out of style with the passing of a single season, we purchase new automobiles in short order—not for their ability to take us somewhere, but to maintain status. And well fitting clothes are not good enough; we have developed the designer jeans mentality. If it is not expensive because of the status conveyed by the label, it is just not worth having. People who suffered through the great depression declared that their children would have everything they did not have. What they did not know was that they were already giving their children the most crucial things that anyone really needs: love, family, and a sense of values. Their children did get many of the material goods their parents lacked, including some unintentional additions: a poor sense of self-worth, a value system based on materialism, drug problems, and high divorce rates.

The designer jeans mentality has taken hold of the entire nation, but it is particularly rampant in the medical profession. A quick trip to your local hospital doctors' parking lot will either leave you amused or angry. Expensive cars with outrageous vanity plates fill the spaces. On late night television, entrepreneurial physicians compete with tasteless used car dealers for advertising time. Clinics flood the media with fancy promotions; mass mailings of slick brochures fill mailboxes; published statistics tell us of the unnecessary procedures performed by physicians. In order to satisfy the desire to pay for the Mercedes or the Jaguar, too many physicians have turned medicine into big business.

Even though only a small portion of doctors display wealth ostentatiously, their actions contribute to the public's negative attitude toward the profession. At one time, the better-than-average salaries of physicians were accepted as fair compensation for heavy responsibility. But now people generally think of physicians with the same disdain they feel for large, impersonal corporations. Unnecessarily large fees are often coupled with a minimum of personal caring for the needs of patients. Far too many of us in the medical profession have been seduced into becoming businessman. We have contributed to making medicine a business and have failed to respond to outside forces which are doing the same.

A first obvious sign of this business orientation is the all too common pattern of overbooking. Physicians try to see too many patients and do not know the word "enough." Some have excellent motivations, not based upon greed. In rural areas, the proportion of doctors to the resident population may cause physicians to feel that they cannot refuse to see patients who need their help. But, as often as not, the motive is financial. Being a dermatologist and a former offender myself, I am keenly aware that some dermatologists run what might politely be called factories of skin care. Over one hundred patients are seen in a day. If a doctor works seven hours a day, patients receive 4.2 minutes of "care" per visit. I have had patients come to me having been deeply offended by the lack of concern and attention they received from my colleagues. One patient complained that he was given only thirty seconds of attention from the physician on his first visit. The patient did not even have an opportunity to ask questions about his complaints. If that wasn't bad enough, on his return visit the doctor was on the phone to his stockbroker and used hand signals to tell the patient to continue on the same medication. The physician never stopped talking to his broker and never said one actual word to the patient who, needless to say, was upset enough to seek a new doctor.

Whatever the motivation a physician might have in overbooking patients, an overworked physician does a disservice to his patients by not being fully present during the office or hospital visit or procedure. Permitting too many patients to be seen in an office day is potentially dangerous.

When physicians contribute to making medicine a business, outside forces move in to capitalize on the situation—literally. A typical example is the establishment of Health Maintenance Organizations (HMOs). These organizations, while promising to lower the cost of health care, in fact, provide profits for administrators and create an atmosphere of moral crisis for participating physicians.

Many physicians join HMOs because of business motivations which have nothing to do with the promotion of excellence in health care. Doctors are afraid that HMOs will take their patients and income away. This was certainly true for me. I joined on the assumption that I would have to recapture some of my lost income, even if it meant getting my former patients back with discounted fees. I held out as long as possible against this new practice, but fear and a need to protect my turf forced me to give in and join. The experience was never satisfying. I have since resigned from all HMOs in which I participated and have discovered an interesting way of filling those patient slots vacated by HMO patients. *Making Medicine Work* is currently developing a project to help other physicians with common views leave HMOs in such a way that their income is only minimally affected.

I joined two types of HMO models. The first was typified by the SHARE HMO in which patients, or their employers, paid monthly premiums to the HMO. The HMO administrators received their salaries and expenses, and what was left of the money was given to primary care physicians with the stipulation that the capitation (or money given to the doctor "per head") was to cover the cost of all physician expenses. If the primary care physician requested a consultation with a specialist, the specialist had to be paid out of the physician's capitation.

It did not take long for the primary care doctors to realize that the less they spent on their patients, the more profit they kept. The number of consultations from certain groups of primary care physicians suddenly reached an all-time low. Some physicians even asked their consultants to "keep the cost down" and cut corners on the care.

One wonders if those primary care physicians whose consultations suddenly dropped were sending too many consultations prior to being part of an HMO or if they suddenly became versed in all specialties and procedures. Considering that a pediatrician takes three years to train, a surgeon five years, a dermatologist three years, an internist three years, an allergist five years, and a urologist five years, the sudden gain in expertise is truly amazing. What happens all too often is that physicians' reimbursement agreements cause them to sacrifice quality of care in order to protect profit.

Excellence in medicine requires that physicians obtain the best for their patients, even if they make less or no money from treating any specific patient. When we perform procedures knowing that someone else could handle them better than ourselves, we offer our patients mediocrity. Physicians may justify their actions with all manner of excuses, but often the truth lies in the realm of income. The moral dilemma of the SHARE model is obvious. Primary care physicians make decisions for their patients with the knowledge, either consciously or subconsciously, that the more they do themselves and the less that is done outside of their offices, the more profit they keep.

The second HMO system I joined is the PRUCARE/MICHAEL REESE HMO. This HMO has full-time salaried primary care doctors available for HMO patients. Specialists are formed into a group which, for a set amount of reimbursement, provides the necessary specialty care for the HMO subscribers.

I joined this HMO after receiving a call from a colleague asking for help. The dermatologist across the street—the very fellow I once envisioned as a bad guy—had refused to continue his participation in this HMO due to slow payment of his fees. Given my dislike of the HMO system, a refusal would have been the most natural response, but I had not as yet experienced my turnaround at that time. My appointment book—the one with far too many slots—was not full. I was being offered a perfect chance to get ahead of my competition; the opportunity looked like a plum, and I was determined to eat it and gloat.

Rather than have empty time in my office, I convinced myself that it would be better to see patients for half my fee, even with the anticipated three to four month delay in payment. My decision was strictly a matter of business, not medicine, but it was a mistake. My office became overloaded with cases primary care doctors should have handled, but because those physicians were on salary, they did not even make an effort to treat the simplest skin problems. They were paid their monthly wages even if they passed their patients on to the specialists.

The HMO had other handicaps. The organization which administered the reimbursement for the specialist group was disorganized. Information and rules changed regularly—with no notice. Patients would show up with little or no advanced warning, and often without their referral forms. The directives on the referral forms were often vague. In order to perform any procedure not identified on the form, I would have to obtain permission from the HMO. My office staff spent valuable time on the telephone—usually on hold—trying to obtain directives from the HMO organization.

The original agreement was that I would give a discount on my regular fee. This was quickly changed when the organization ran short of funds. Specialists were given a maximum sum they could earn, no matter how much work they did. After a certain number of office visits per month, I was essentially giving free care to HMO patients. Though I was bound and determined to give part of my practice to the poor, I did not consider most HMO patients as qualifying for charity. My resentment of HMOs grew as my office became overloaded with patients whose most basic complaints should have been handled by the salaried primary care physicians.

It is normal human behavior to desire rewards for effort expended. When treating public aid or charity patients for free, the rewards exceed the

money that could have been earned. The satisfaction obtained is a pleasure that no amount of
money can replace. Subscribers to an HMO,
however, are not charity patients. What I was
doing was supporting the administration of the
HMO and giving my time and services to patients
who, for the most part, could afford the visits.
These patients should have been cared for by the
salaried doctors on staff who were receiving
most of the compensation. As long as my time
was being given away for free, I decided to give
it to those people who could not afford it, and I
dropped out of the HMO system.

Making my decision to remove myself from all
participation in HMO medicine meant losing the
income earned from seeing those patients. At a
certain point, however, money becomes secondary to one's integrity. My office staff backed me
in my decision; in fact, they wanted to vote me
physician employer of the year. Ending participation in HMOs freed them from endless
phone calls, hassles, and the need to be familiar
with the constantly changing ground rules for
the different systems in which we participated.

My decision to leave the HMO system was
based on my commitment to excellence in
patient care. With my eyes now open, I noticed
patterns of patient behavior which were disturbing. Some patients came to see me only in crisis
situations. I came to realize that some of these

patients had failed to show up at office visits, often without calling to cancel. When I took the time to talk and listen to them, I was surprised to learn that a large percentage of them had been avoiding care for lack of money. Many of them were too embarrassed to discuss their financial situations. Others said they didn't even consider the possibility that fees could be reduced to an affordable level. In most of these cases, the patients would have benefited from regular checkups. It certainly would have been wiser had they come to see me when problems began to flair, rather than waiting for them to become serious.

Now when I find one of these patients in my practice, I reduce my fees to an affordable amount. Sometimes, a few dollars can make the difference for the patient. These small amounts of money, in the long run, do not make any significant difference in my income. Patients who realize that they can afford the visits take greater responsibility with regard to their follow-up office visits, and they feel less threatened by medical problems. The patients are also responsible for letting me know if their financial situation changes either way, whether they can pay fully or if additional support is needed. This system runs on patient honor. These individuals have been my patients for years; I have neither the time nor inclination to do formal financial screenings. Eventually, someone will be seen for less money than they should be paying. But I believe in people's basic honesty. Patients who are dishonest with me will have to live with their own consciences.

Within my practice, my intention is to fill those appointments vacated by HMO patients with my own patients, paying discounted fees. It is a process by which both the patients and I win. Patients win because they receive excellent health care at an affordable price. They no longer need to wait until they are in trouble to seek my help, and they take greater responsibility for their own health. Waiting until a crisis develops is false economy: extra tests and medications are often required and infected skin irritations may require costly antibiotics.

I win by filling empty appointment times with patients paying discounted fees equal to the amounts paid by HMOs, but paid at the time of service by grateful patients. Furthermore, HMO patients have little or no choice in deciding which physicians will treat them; my private patients choose to see me. My office is no longer saddled with additional paperwork or phone calls. Former HMO patients are welcome to continue to see me. They must, however, pay for their own care. To my delight and surprise, some of them have chosen to do so.

Looking outward from my practice, I realized that people who couldn't quite afford the cost of health care were everywhere. Surprisingly, most of these people are not poor; the poor generally are covered by public aid, but workers often do not qualify for such help. Families with young children often live from paycheck to paycheck, scraping by on necessities. When they try to budget by eliminating medical expenses, the consequences can be painful and injurious to health. As I began talking with my fellow physicians, I found that many of them were willing to replace HMO patients with such patients, even at reduced fees.

A common concern of physicians I spoke with was that, while they were willing to help patients themselves, they feared what might happen if hospitalization were required. When I began to look into the matter, I found that most of these patients are covered by some form of hospitalization insurance. For those who are not, hospitalization policies with high deductibles are available at reasonable costs. Through a program called the Star Project©, we are now encouraging patients to purchase such policies, with the understanding that certain physicians will reduce office fees during those years in which families are getting on their feet financially.

Making Medicine Work, Inc. is currently sponsoring a pilot project which will financially qualify those members of our community with lower incomes who would seek regular health care if they received a reduced fee. The processing will be done by social service personnel. Patients will be placed on a sliding fee scale. Doctors may access this bank of pre-qualified patients and take as many as fit into their practices.

Doctors accepting these patients instead of HMO patients would find an easy way to maintain their incomes and eliminate the problems of HMO medicine. Young physicians in practice who have available time and a less than full practice could accept a number of these patients. Many of the patients are upwardly mobile young families who will not need reduced fees forever. They will certainly be grateful and loyal to any physician who assisted them when support was required.

The project is not without cost and would require funding for the social service personnel and administration. Patients and physicians will be charged a fee to enter this program, but the fees would be minimal and would only cover the cost of the administration; the setup, in other words, would be basically not-for-profit.

In spite of the fears of many physicians, there is really no scarcity of patients who need medical help. A lack of either money or the courage to ask for a reduction in fees keeps many would-be patients away from our offices. Were doctors to lower their fees for patients who needed help, their offices would never be empty.

The interference from private "cost reducing" enterprises is not the only threat to the quality of health care. Doctors already feel the hand of government interference in the Medicare system. Hospital stays are cut short and certain treatments are dictated by government managers in the name of cost containment, a cost control which often decreases the quality of care. Patients are commonly sent home from a hospital earlier than is prudent because a clerk in Washington follows guidelines and regulations without regard to the patient—a human being.

Because we, as physicians, have directly made and indirectly allowed medicine to be made into a big business, we are vulnerable to being bought out by anyone with the nerve to buy into the business. Government and corporate America are doing just that, and we are standing idly by during the takeover. We wring our hands and bemoan our fate, not realizing that we have the power to shape and mold medicine into whatever we wish it to be. Nothing is being taken from us that we are not giving away ourselves.

The irony about the takeovers of medicine is that for the most part, the public does not approve of them. Although our profession has its critics who look for every opportunity to discredit us, the public still would like to support us. They want choices regarding who they see for their medical care and the treatments they receive. Health care providers and patients share the same fear that we will all be forced into a government system in which nobody has any say in running the system except bureaucrats.

The general conditions of the medical profession in recent years have created much dissatisfaction amongst physicians. Most are resigned to seeing American medicine falling prey to outside control and they despair of the possibility of initiating meaningful change. The emotions in discussions on the subject vary from sadness and disgust to anger. Doctors' visions of the future are bleak. Too many physicians have become resigned to the inevitability of a government takeover of American medicine, though they feel that socialized medicine would be a final blow to excellence in the treatment of patients.

Some doctors stop short of taking any action to improve the medical environment because they feel overwhelmed and powerless against a problem which seems bigger than they are. Others are stopped because they have something to lose. If doctors become too verbal about medicine and its problems, they stand to lose referrals from their fellow physicians and a sizable portion of future income. For physicians whose entire clientele comes from referrals from primary care doctors, this threat may be very real indeed. I would argue that it is time for physicians to become vocal. To those physicians who have resisted the lure of materialism, I would urge you to do your part in reclaiming the integrity of the profession, and let your community know what you are doing. While physicians remain silent, they share the responsibility for allowing the more verbal business-oriented doctors to create the image of medicine that now exists in the public eye.

Those of us who are trying to make medicine work cannot afford the luxury of self-satisfaction. We cannot be afraid our colleagues will think us strange to shun the modern business-oriented side of medicine. We need to unify and support each other until the world starts to see that the majority of us are truly dedicated to our patients and our profession. Our fellow physicians must learn about the true satisfaction in medicine which we receive from practicing selflessly.

Many physicians I have talked to have argued that what we do cannot change medicine, that the problems are out of control. To them I answer: *we are medicine*, and what we say and do about it is what it is. By saying nothing, we surrender our rights to determine the future for ourselves and the nation.

My patients have interesting reactions when I explain my personal transformation and that my office has been changed to emphasize a total commitment to excellence in patient care. Many of them tell me how rare it is to find a doctor who believes in the concept, much less practices it. I know I am not alone in practicing this way. But although I am not, too many people out there believe that what I am doing is unusual.

When physicians take their responsibilities seriously, they resemble the doctors I remember from my childhood. Offices do not become factories of medicine in which too many patients are seen in a day. Patients are no longer sent directly to emergency rooms because physicians are too busy with social events. What is missing in the medical profession today is the former total commitment to patient care. At one time, a life spent in medicine was a life dedicated to long hours and selfless service to patients. Doctors surely had to be concerned about making enough money to run their offices and support their families, but for a majority of physicians, that financial concern was secondary. When they became doctors, they gave up the rights to certain freedoms and, in turn, were granted status, privileges and a high level of income.

Society tolerated physicians having comfortable incomes and a high social status because, by the way they were practicing, doctors were making a contribution to society. In the past, doctors who would treat first and worry about getting paid later were easy to find. Doctors accrued large amounts of accounts receivable, knowing that they would probably never be paid the entire amount. Even so, they received enough income to live better than most of their patients. They took a great deal from the world, but gave even more back.

It is my mostly deeply held personal belief that the best way for physicians to improve the quality of medical care in the country is to take part in a 'ground up' reform of American medicine. If we take control of our own profession, the temptation for corporations and the government to usurp our functions will diminish. What will be necessary to regain the faith and support of the public? A sense of reasonable sacrifice. If we can keep the designer jeans, Mercedes mentality in check, we will be able to live well without promoting resentment and jealousy.

My recommendations are simple:

1. If physicians everywhere contributed a portion of their time to charity, patients would once again come to see that we put their needs first. I do not contend that all physicians must follow the models I am using. Local conditions vary,

and different approaches can be used in different areas. The point, however, is simple. If a community feels that its physicians practice for the benefit of all its members, everyone benefits.

2. We must treat our patients as if they are important to us; this requires offering every patient adequate time, not only to treat ills but also to educate in wise health practices, as well as listening when a sympathetic ear is needed.

The kind of care which would be offered is the type which in the past won respect for the medical profession. Patients, incidentally, are far less likely to sue someone they love and respect, someone who is recognized as a contributor to a community's well-being. As the nation has gained in wealth, we have too often lost the sense of community—of sharing in common goals and mutual support. It is possible to make the recommended contribution without giving up a comfortable lifestyle. The choice does not have to be made between becoming an Albert Schweitzer or a Donald Trump.

Section II

THE EDUCATED PATIENT

In the ultimate depth of being, we find ourselves no longer separate but, rather, part of the unity of the universe. That unity includes the sufferer and the suffering, and the healer and that which heals. Therefore, all acts of healing are ultimately our selves healing our Self.

Ram Dass
"The Intuitive Heart"
From **Healers on Healing**

Remove all pedestals from beneath people. Those who stand tall do it on their own.

Personal Communication
Bernie Siegel, M. D.

Chapter III

UNDERSTANDING WELLNESS

We have all seen it on TV: the ad in which a bedraggled and dispirited cold sufferer has been overwhelmed by those horrible cold and flu symptoms we all experience occasionally: sore throat, runny nose, headache, and fever. Then comes the inevitable contrasting scene: moments after taking whatever product is being advertised, the same individual is off to work or play, totally free of all symptoms and as smiley as a kid in a candy store. It is little wonder that as a nation we are poorly educated regarding issues of health and disease. And it is even more obvious why we are a society on drugs: we are

57

endlessly told that pain and distress can be removed and replaced with happiness via a magic pill—a chemical concoction. The prevalence of such commercials suggests that generally accepted ideas regarding health and disease are often distortions.

The type of advertisement just alluded to is based on a false implication, namely that symptoms of disease and disease are one and the same thing. While such advertisements sometimes admit that the product is merely intended to relieve symptoms, the upbeat mood and tone suggest that the cold sufferer has been cured of his malady and is free to return to normal activities. But going about one's business in normal fashion shortly after the onset of a viral infection is probably the least wise course of action.

Let us examine briefly what happens when one contracts a cold virus. The invading pathogen, the virus, takes up residence in the body's cells in places in which it can thrive: the mucous membranes of the sinuses, the throat, and sometimes even the lungs. The resultant irritation will produce the redness and soreness evident in a physical inspection of the throat; swelling may occur in the sinuses, the pressure of which can produce a headache; the nose will begin to run as the body attempts to flush away the pathogen; and fever will develop as the body's immune system fights the virus. The over-the-counter drug may bring temporary relief from some of these symptoms, but it does not cure the cold sufferer of the disease; it does not, in other words, destroy the offending pathogen. A symptom, after all, is a manifestation of the body's attempt to defend itself. In effect, what you have purchased is a dose of something that can do absolutely no good in freeing you from the underlying cause of your cold. Will you feel better? Maybe. But if you do and you proceed to go to work or school as such ads suggest you can do in comfort (and where, incidentally, you can infect a lot of other people who will then buy the same type of medication), you may actually become even more sick because you will not be giving your body the advantage it needs to fight the pathogen—namely rest. Therefore, the wisdom of suppressing the symptoms is questionable, especially since suppression is not a cure, and the illusion of being cured may increase your chances of becoming more sick.

Let's take the logic a step further. An individual has a cold which is a real knockout. The condition is much worse than usual, and the individual decides to see a doctor. The diagnosis in layman's terms is a bad cold, and the doctor issues a prescription for an antibiotic. The patient goes home and follows the physician's instructions: gets plenty of bed rest and takes the antibiotic down to the last pill. Ten days later he is completely cured. Can the doctor take credit for the healing? Not really. An antibiotic has absolutely no effect on the various viruses which are responsible for the common cold. The doctor is aware of this. If he prescribed an antibiotic, he probably did so because individuals suffering from bad colds often develop secondary bacterial infections, commonly in the sinuses or lungs. He may issue the antibiotic as a preventive against such infection or because a bacterial infection has already taken hold. Or he may issue the antibiotic just because patients expect to be given something when they pay for medical help. Although an antibiotic will help the body's immune system destroy bacteria, the bacteria were not the cause of the cold in the first place. Infective bacteria are a totally different type of pathogen than are viruses. Why does the cold go away then? Because the human immune system eventually destroys the virus. What is the point of all this? It is simple: the human body insofar as it is cured tends to cure itself. All medications are merely intended to be aids to this functioning. Patients too often do not understand what a doctor can do for them and what they should be doing for themselves to promote their own health.

From years of discussing the practice of medicine with professional colleagues, I can safely say that the public in general tends to expect that physicians should be healers who can magically solve patients' problems with an injection, pill, or operative procedure. However spectacular the accomplishments of modern medicine are, what doctors do is never magical. In fact, I would venture to say that the more miraculous a procedure seems to be, the less likely it is to be prudent and safe. An example: an individual with extreme reactions to seasonal pollens goes to a doctor and gets an "allergy shot" which clears up the "problem" over an extended period of time. The uninformed patient is relieved of the troubling symptoms, feels wonderful, and talks with admiration about the "allergy" injection. But the patient also does not understand the potential consequences of the procedure; normally if a patient is given only one injection, he has received a long-term cortisone shot, which suppresses the human immune system, the very system which protects the body from disease. Good physicians administer such shots only with the greatest of caution and never in routine fashion or on a regular basis, year after year during allergy season. The alternate procedure for treating allergy problems requires a long series of injections of minute amounts of the allergen which gradually desensitize the patient to it. Although not always successful, this safer procedure takes time and careful monitoring by an allergist. Another example: a deeply depressed individual seeks medical help and is given a drug to alleviate depression. The drug is effective, so effective in fact that the patient eventually becomes drug dependent. While I concede that there are various specific types of mental illness in which chemical interruption becomes necessary to allow an individual to function (paranoid schizophrenia, for example), far too often physicians can create drug dependence by not taking the time and showing the necessary concern to help an emotionally disturbed individual. In many cases the best help would be reference to another health professional who has wider experience in dealing with psychological problems.

What are the practical implications of what I am saying? Don't put physicians on pedestals and expect that whatever you do to yourself, they can solve your problems. Instead take responsibility for your own health, promote it every day in the way you live, and when you do become ill, learn to ask intelligent questions of your physician.

Individual responsibility is the key to wellness. If your body says that you have a vicious flu or cold, don't take a medication to suppress the symptoms and then assume you can function in normal fashion. While over-the-counter drugs may make you feel momentarily better, you still are ill and if you act irresponsibly, you may get worse. If you have a really bad cold or flu, get a day or two of bed rest. Many people would protest: but my job is too important for me to miss work. Really? Better to miss a day or two now than five later. Will your firm really benefit if you spread the cold to a half dozen other workers?

Health is your responsibility. Every individual should take sensible steps to promote and preserve health. Some of these steps are painfully obvious: don't smoke and don't abuse alcohol or drugs. If you are already trapped in bad habits, seek help, professional help if necessary, to change your behavior. Just exactly what you should eat and how much you should exercise may be slightly more complicated issues, depending on your age and physical condition. But for most people, common sense can serve as a guide. The issue of just how much cholesterol an egg yolk contains is probably not as important to your well-being as is eating a balanced diet. Not much has really changed since I was a child when the popular wisdom was "eat your vegetables and go easy on the candy." If you are overweight and you need to reduce, do not take up any fad diets which will deprive you of necessary nutrients and thereby endanger your health. You should still eat well—although less—and you should lose some of the weight through increased exercise. While jogging or swimming or bicycling may be appropriate for many individuals, almost everyone can benefit from a brisk walk. It is beyond the scope of this book to cover issues of nutrition and exercise, but scientifically sound information on such subjects is readily available in virtually any library.

What individuals everywhere should strive for is what I call wellness. Being well does not necessarily mean that you will not become sick. It does mean that you take care of your body in such a way that when you do face an illness, your body will be best able to respond because you have maintained its well-being at optimal efficiency.

The human body is an amazingly complex mechanism. During every hour of the night and day, your brain and hormonal system work nonstop to keep your body chemistry in balance. Quite apart from you making any conscious effort, your body works to establish and maintain the equilibrium which allows you to live in health. And most of the time, it is successful; the normal condition of life is to be healthy. Generally, it takes just a little common sense and self-discipline to maintain good health, given the amazing powers of the body to keep itself well, to fight pathogens, and to recuperate from disease or injury.

But disease and accidents do occur. While we are made to be well, no one can maintain health all the time. And, of course, we are mortal; we must die. Being well, I would argue, includes these recognitions: the power of our bodies to keep us in good health, provided we treat them reasonably, and the realization that we cannot be free of disease or death. What makes us well? Largely an attitude toward what we are: an active concern for living in healthy fashion and an acceptance of the conditions which are unavoidable. Physicians are well aware of the fact that among patients who are seriously ill, attitude has much to do with their ability to recuperate. A positive attitude seems to maximize the body's chances of healing itself. Even terminally ill patients will often surprise physicians, not merely by their ability to delay death, but by the grace with which they accept their illness and by the ability to function above norms.

Being well is, in my opinion, being able to love and to accept love, no matter what the condition of the body is. Even a person dying of terminal cancer can be well if the individual is able to accept the condition without resentment and is still able to show love and concern to one's fellow man. If you think back over your own past, you will probably be able to remember a time when a disease seemed to be much worse than normal because the physical problem was coupled with resentment, hatred, frustration or undue pressures. Conversely, a person who can accept the inevitability of occasional illnesses and who deals with them with equanimity will normally seem to be less seriously ill and will recuperate more quickly and fully.

Physicians can help you when problems, serious or otherwise, develop, but they cannot live your life for you. They cannot make the day-to-day decisions about how you live, what stress you put yourself under, what you eat, and how much exercise you get. Doctors will have their pills and their procedures—most of which can be used prudently and effectively. But you should be informed about what makes you healthy, what keeps you well, and what steps are prudent in recovering from diseases.

Chapter IV

DOCTOR AND PATIENT AS PARTNERS

In defense of my profession, I will begin with an assertion: the overwhelming majority of health care workers practicing today are well-trained and committed to patient welfare. A problem arises because we tend to hear more—and talk more—about the exceptions. This chapter will be designed to help you find the excellent health care professionals and to get the most out of what they can offer you. There is no need to settle for a doctor or other professional who is second rate.

67

To develop a clear understanding of the issue of medicine, let us begin with a consideration of what it means to be a healer. I am not referring only to medical doctors. At times, problems can be resolved more readily by other health care professionals. Take my childhood headaches, for example. Expensive tests administered by experts were unable to turn up any satisfactory explanation of their cause. I suffered them until I outgrew a need for them. No physician was able to offer an adequate recommendation. However, had someone else, a social worker or a psychologist, been able to see that I generated the headaches in response to tension and out of self-pity, I might have been cured of my problem. A healer is anyone who can promote wellness, whether the individual is a physician, nurse, social worker, psychologist, chiropractor, or acupuncturist.

I have already suggested that individuals must take responsibility for their own wellness by promoting their health on a day-to-day basis. Let us now consider the role of a healer in helping an individual who becomes ill. Ideally the relationship of healer and patient should be a partnership. If the patient has not put the healer on a pedestal and shifted responsibility away from the self, then the patient and healer can enter a cooperative arrangement to help the person who is ill—not merely to recover from a temporary illness, but to promote wellness on a regular basis.

I quite often hear patients complaining about other doctors, contending that they were not cured because a physician failed to give them the right medicine. Such assertions remind me of the magic pill mentality. I usually try to spend some time explaining to complaining patients that the fault may not lie with the physician but with them. I ask questions like: Did you ask about the possibility of alternate medications or approaches? Did you accurately and carefully identify your symptoms? Did you hide any information out of fear? Did you follow the physician's advice carefully and take your medication as directed? And the most important question of all: have you made an effort to promote wellness on a regular basis or are you expecting a doctor to cure you no matter what you do to yourself? Doctors and patients cannot afford to be working at odds with one another. A physician can do most for a patient who works at maintaining health.

Let us now look at what ideally should happen during a visit to a healer by first considering what type of problems often occur during visitations. I can assert unequivocally from years of experience that the underlying causes of virtually all problems stem from a lack of adequate communication between healer and patient. The fault can lie with either party. Oftentimes physicians are so heavily overworked that they will assume total control of a diagnosis and make the patient feel as if he or she has no role in the process of being cured. Obviously, this is a bad situation; physicians and other health professionals should understand that patients who are treated as if their actions can contribute to their well-being will have a higher likelihood of following advice. Healers should avoid treating patients like dehumanized problems or mere pill receptacles.

Medical practitioners who are first rate all have excellent listening skills. They will often be sensitive enough to "fill in the gaps" in what the patient is saying, either by sensing that a patient is suppressing information out of fear or by knowing pathology well enough to interpret statements wisely and to ask insightful follow-up questions. All healers, in addition to being good listeners, should answer all questions clearly and honestly. And they should take the time necessary to explain a diagnosis, the recommended procedure for promoting recovery, and the potential problems or side affects which might accompany any therapeutic regimen. Anything short of that ideal is a failure of communication.

I also believe that a physician, or indeed any health practitioner, should discuss alternate forms of therapy for individuals who may benefit from seeing a health professional with a different speciality. Sometimes a psychologist or chiropractor will be able to help an individual more than a physician can; and, of course, the reverse is also true: at times any speciality is liable to be too limited for the problem at hand. Patients should also be given a chance to discuss alternate, non-traditional, healing strategies, especially if surgery is a recommended procedure. Physicians should be willing to offer solid information on what the success rates, or lack thereof, are for alternate approaches to healing.

The failure of adequate communication can also be the fault of the patient. Quite commonly a patient will suppress information out of fear. It is simple human nature not to want to confront frightening news. I have had the experience: a sudden new pain convinces me that something very serious is wrong with me, and the natural reaction is not to want to have someone look into it. When the pain disappears in a day or two and I realize it was nothing more than a stiff muscle, I feel at once relieved and slightly foolish. But sometimes strange new aches are warnings of serious problems, and one thing we do know about medicine is that a very significant proportion of life-threatening diseases like cancer can be controlled *if* early detection leads to early treatment. Overcome those fears, and do not be afraid of seeming foolish. There is no such thing as a dumb question; where your health is concerned, the only foolish thing you can do is to totally ignore any warning sign of potential disease. When you ask a question about a pain or a problem, only a few responses are likely and most of them are good. If your problem is insignificant medically, you will have set your fears to rest. And the healer will certainly feel good about relieving your anxiety. If a problem is serious, detection is far better than ignorance. Early detection and control are the secrets of increased longevity and quality of life.

Another problem which any patient should face up to is the problem of money. For many Americans, a visit to a physician can be a burden, even at times a prohibitive expense. I honestly believe if patients were forthright about such problems—admittedly difficult to discuss because of embarrassment—most physicians would make every effort to accommodate patients' needs, either by offering to defer payment in installments, or reducing fees, or eliminating them altogether for the specific visit. In fact, most physicians would probably feel better in knowing that a fee will be paid in, for instance, two installments on the first of the month than to worry about all the bills that are not being paid, privately resenting patients who will not admit that payment is a burden. Patients would also feel more at ease and be less inclined to avoid their physicians because of the embarrassment of having defaulted on earlier payments, thereby putting off examinations until a crisis arises. Be honest with your physicians, and they will almost certainly do what they can to help you.

Which brings me the other side of the coin: the patient's responsibility in the partnership—it is a reciprocal relationship, after all. If you make an appointment, you should show up for it, on time. Most physicians cannot afford to wait around for a patient who is late; they have busy schedules. I am acutely aware of this now that I have far fewer patient slots than I once did. If several patients miss appointments in one day, I end up wasting time which could be used productively in helping someone else. Patients need to grant the same respect to physicians that they give to United Airlines. Would you show up an hour late at the airport and expect a flight to be held for you? And if you do have to wait to see a physician, try to complain only if you are being rushed in the office. If the physician is listening and coaching you well, understand that delays may be the result of everyone being treated conscientiously.

And individuals who can afford to pay for a visit should pay on time—that is, when the services are rendered. In case the general public is not aware of it, doctors and medical professionals face one of the highest rates of nonpayment or late payment from patrons. Yes, physicians' fees can seem to be high, but a medical office or a clinic is not an inexpensive business to run. Doctors must pay their nurses and secretaries; they must retire debts on medical offices and clinics, in addition to paying astronomical malpractice fees. Young physicians may also be paying off debts from medical school. I suppose that non-paying members of the public assume that all physicians are rich and therefore capable of absorbing non-payment of fees. First of all, that is not true; many physicians, especially those who have been in the profession for less than ten years are liable to have negative net worth. Besides, the consequences of non-payment are obvious, as my own history attests. When you don't pay your physicians on time, you force them to become more, not less, money oriented. If you are not paying, they have to worry about taking on more patients to generate sufficient income, and you contribute to the erosion of the quality of health care. Give physicians at least the respect you show an automobile repair shop. When you have your automobile fixed, you don't get your keys back until you write the check. You shouldn't expect doctors will see you for free, not unless they assent to doing so upon mutual agreement.

Here then, in capsule form, are my rules for making the most of an office visit.

1. Be comfortable with your doctor or healer as a professional committed to your well-being. If he or she appears to be more interested in you as a dollar sign, or if you do not get answers to your questions because you are being unduly rushed, or if the physician assumes that you do not need to know about your own health, look around for another physician. There are lots of wonderful doctors who do care.

2. When you go to see a physician, be prepared to discuss the reasons for your visit. If you are ill, identify your symptoms thoroughly. Organize your thoughts and do not hesitate to include any information which you think may be medically significant. Also prepare a list of questions about your condition; patients often forget to ask questions and then phone the physician after the visit is over. Obviously being prepared is a better strategy and shows courtesy to the doctor by not interrupting him when he is helping his subsequent patients. Doctors are quite willing to be interrupted if a problem arises, but patient thoughtfulness can make a physician's job easier.

3. While in most cases you will defer to the physician's expertise, you want to have faith and confidence in what he recommends, and you can do this most effectively if you educate yourself—both in and out of the office—about your general health and any problems which you may face. If

you are certain a diagnosis is wrong, do not hesitate to seek a second opinion.

4. In the office, be prepared to listen as well as talk. If a physician talks in language which is obscure to you, politely ask for a clarification. And don't let anxiety shut down your listening ability. Commonly when I announce that I will be administering an injection, patients will stop listening and begin anticipating the discomfort of the needle. Keep your ears open. Good physicians want you to understand what is wrong with you and what you have to do to promote healing. If you fail to follow their instructions—and a stunningly high percentage of patients ignore their physician's advice—the doctor is almost certain to see you again, most often when you are in a foul and accusatory mood.

5. Follow your physician's instructions. When a medication is prescribed, you should ask about the exact purpose and function of the medication and what possible side effects you are likely to experience. Be sure you know how you can reach the physician or someone who is on call in the event any unforeseen problems arise.

6. While you should feel free to ask as many questions as are necessary to clarify the physician's diagnosis and recommended regimen, do not waste the physician's time with small talk. If stories about your relatives are not

important to the diagnosis, invite the physician to hear them after work on Friday. If the stories are interesting, your doctor will probably be happy to hear them away from the office.

7. Be responsible and a good partner. Expect that your physician will be personally concerned about you, but also work at maintaining your health by following recommendations conscientiously. Most importantly, do not put off visits until a situation deteriorates and then ask for magical remedies. Be sensitive to your body. There are a number of good, relatively inexpensive books available which list symptoms and when their characteristics dictate that you should have them checked by a physician.

The vision I have for medicine in the future is based on a transformation of the health care system. Individuals will take primary responsibility for their own health. Whether we want to be or not, each of us is responsible for the consequences of our own actions. As a nation we need to take the credit card mentality out of medicine. It is too easy nowadays for a person to say, "Heck, I'll keep smoking. If I develop emphysema later, the government will pay for my treatment." What would happen if everyone had to pay for their treatments out of their own pockets first? Perhaps we would be wiser and take better care of ourselves. If you abuse your body, neglect it, or ignore it, you won't get another one. It is yours. The miracles of modern medicine are such that you may be able to get another heart, but is that really what you want? Health is worth pursuing on a daily basis so that you will not need extreme measures merely to be able to survive.

When illness does strike, and it is unavoidable, the patient turns to the physician or other health professional for help. But patients must recognize that their doctors are not magicians. Lest I give a wrong impression, I acknowledge that we do have excellent drugs, some justifiably called miracle drugs. Antibiotics, for example, have saved untold lives which a mere fifty years ago would have been lost—and how often those lives were children's lives. But doctors, armed with their pharmaceuticals and procedures, should not be thought of as having supernatural powers. The proper role of a physician is much like that of a coach. Doctors can diagnose disease and recommend the most beneficial course of action; they can prescribe medication, but the patient is the player who must follow the recommendations and execute the plan. And one of the most significant strategies a patient can have is to practice prevention. Work at being healthy.

Here is a checklist which will be helpful for your visits to the doctor:

1. Do you have a list of questions that you have prepared in advance?

2. Are you on time for your visit? If your doctor is a specialist who is often called out of the office on emergency calls, it might be in your interest to call first before leaving your home.

3. Do you have a list of medications you are currently taking, including names and dosages?

4. Do you have a list of any allergies you might have, especially to medication?

5. Are you aware of the doctor's policies regarding payment and insurance? Does the doctor accept public aid or Medicare?

6. How can you reach the doctor in case of an emergency? How fast is the response time? What hours are the office open (evenings, etc.)? How easy is it to call and have your questions answered? Will the doctor call you back, if needed, and how long will that generally take?

7. Are you hiding any information or fears from your doctor?

8. Are you prepared to be honest with your doctor regarding use of alcohol, recreational drugs, and safe sex practices?

9. Are you willing to accept your doctor as a partner and not as the person with the "magic cures"?

Doctor's checklist:

1. Have you handled your personal problems for the day so you can be mentally fresh and available for your patients?

2. If you have seen this patient before, are you aware of the patient's problems? Can you review the chart prior to the visit?

3. At the start of the visit, do you give the patient space to re-establish a relationship with you, or do you immediately start to discuss the medical issues?

4. Is there a dialogue between you and the patient, or do you do all the talking, not encouraging the patient to express his or her fears?

5. Do you make sure you ask the patients about any other problems you feel they might be hiding, or are too shy to talk about?

6. Do you clearly state what responsibility you will take in the care of the patient and what the patient's responsibility is?

7. When giving instructions, do you check that the patient understands them by making the patient repeat them back to you? Do you use

appropriate written handouts to reinforce your instructions?

8. Do you speak in plain English with as little medical jargon as possible?

9. Do you make suggestions for change in non-judgmental ways, or do you impose your value system on the patient?

10. Do you inform patients of the major side effects of all medications and be sure to check any current medications (including over-the-counter) they might be taking?

11. Do you allow enough time for patients to feel comfortable and not rushed?

12. Do you allow yourself to be disturbed with phone calls (except for emergencies) when you are with patients?

13. Are you aware of the patient's lifestyle and any problems the patient might have with following your prescribed treatment?

14. Are you having fun each day and leaving some time for yourself?

Section III

TECHNOLOGY

Healing is letting go of our fear of the concept of death, and recognizing that our true reality is a spiritual one—with no limitations. Healing means letting go of the concept that our identity is limited to a personality and a body that is doomed sooner or later to be hurt, be rejected, get sick, and die.

Gerald Jampolsky
"Living and Loving One Second At A Time"
From *Healers On Healing*

The greatest task before civilization at present is to make machines what they ought to be, the slaves instead of the masters of men.

Havelock Ellis

Chapter V

THE PROBLEM AT ITS SOURCE

Technology. The word defines a modern industrial society's approach to problem solving. When we face problems—a need for increased energy or food resources—we tend to look for technological solutions, which are almost always perceived as being progressive and good. Try, for example, to name a twentieth century advancement that is not tied to technology. The influence of technology is even felt in the arts; in music, for example, innovation is coming from the creation and manipulation of sound via computer simulation.

Technology has played an important role in medical advances. The development in this century of X-rays, electron microscopes, CT scans, and a myriad of other devices has contributed to an ever growing understanding of the human body. By discovering the structure of the individual human cell with its component parts and interrelationships, science has made great progress in identifying how a healthy body works and why and how disease disrupts the body's normal processes. In addition, science has developed what I call the "high visibility" side of technological medicine, the advances which receive lots of attention in the media: heart and organ transplants, and developments like laser surgery.

All these achievements are certainly impressive, but they are also financially costly and they thus contribute to the upward spiral of medical costs. But I would like to hold off discussing economics until the next chapter and point out something that is often overlooked regarding technology: namely, that an emphasis on technological solutions can be costly, not only in monetary, but also in human terms.

When I was in my first year of post-graduate medical training, a year of pediatrics, one of my patients was a sixteen year old boy who was dying of leukemia. Because he would often experience great pain or go through low periods, I

spent a great deal of time with him. We spent
many long nights together and grew to be quite
close. I learned a lot about living and dying from
this young man—and about courage.

Regrettably, no cure had as yet been developed
for leukemia, nor were the advances which have
been made in recent years foreseen at the time.
Nowadays 75 percent of childhood leukemia is
curable; at that time, the process by which white
blood cells multiply uncontrollably was considered irreversible. The primary technique
which was being used to try to help the boy was
to administer periodic blood transfusions to
prolong life. The disease, however, takes a
frightful toll as the end nears. Pain and suffering
increase and strength is lost. As my young friend
was losing his battle, nobly I might say, I was
called to his side one night to help him through
a particularly rough period. We talked all night
long. The boy confessed to me that he had no
fear of death, that he was resigned to its inevitability, and that he wanted me to ask the
physicians in charge to stop the transfusions
which were only prolonging his painful condition. I commiserated with him and promised
that I would try to intervene. Though I made an
impassioned appeal to the doctors in charge, they
categorically refused to accede to the boy's
wishes. Had the transfusions been cut off, the
end would have been reasonably quick, and the

boy could have been spared much continued suffering. Making a patient comfortable and allowing him to die with dignity is not a complex challenge for modern medicine, at least not for the short term. As it turns out, he continued to be given transfusions for three to four more agonizing weeks. I spent many hours with him during that time, and I can tell you that none of them were easy—I felt as if I had failed him. When the end did approach, and it did not come swiftly, he sent out an appeal for his doctors to come to his bedside. Though the message was given to everyone who had treated him, I was the only one to show up for the agonizing last hours. Those doctors who had imposed technological solutions on that brave kid were not there.

You can imagine the profound effect that the experience had on me. It made me question the whole medical school experience and how soon-to-be doctors were being trained. Technology was being used, but not well. A human spirit was being crushed, not simply because technology was being used, but because human beings made bad and self-serving judgments regarding how it should be used.

I will go further in placing at least some of the blame of problems we face on the medical school experience. In the old days of the Doctor Becks, making rounds in a hospital meant visiting the patient to discuss the progress of recovery. Vital signs were checked and progress charts studied, but the analysis was always based on concern for the individual human being. In medical school, we commonly made "rounds" in a conference room, aided not by what any patient might say but only by the statistical information which could be collected from various monitoring devices, from the simple thermometer to extremely sophisticated machines. To me, this tendency to leave the patient and his thoughts, feelings, and pains out of diagnostic evaluations was a form of dehumanization. The assumption which underlies such treatment is that health is a matter of technically controlling microbes and tissue without reference to the fact that they are part of a larger system which affects a real life. I firmly believe that when patients are thought of in such detached fashion, physicians are one step away from seeing humans as dollar signs.

Although some positive changes have been made in recent years, I am still painfully aware of the lack of a real concern for the human side of medicine in most medical schools. It was typical for me to go right from a class on bones and muscles and tissue to a session in clinical practice. Emphasis was never given to the human side of medicine. Some of the most important concerns of being a good doctor—for example, learning to sense a patient's fear and

89

resultant silence regarding symptoms—were never even broached as topics, much less discussed.

My position on this issue is simple. I firmly believe that from the first day of medical school, a commitment must be made to educate and train the whole physician, not merely offer the technical knowledge necessary to be proficient. In no way am I saying that we should lower standards regarding the mastery of the technical details of science and medicine. A doctor must know his field and he must know how to do research when rare and unusual cases confront him as they inevitably confront every physician. He must also be committed to a lifelong process of learning, given the constant growth of medical knowledge. But what good does it do a patient if a doctor commands all the knowledge in the world but cannot communicate effectively with the patient? What good did it do the boy with leukemia? He could not communicate his feelings to the doctors because they would not even confront him, having made their technical choices about his fate in the safety of a conference room.

Some may argue that it is not possible to teach ethics. Maybe it isn't; maybe values are learned by example. But if that is true, think of how much young medical students could benefit by seeing a caring and astute physician make rounds on patients who are actually suffering and in need, not only of treatments, but of moral support. Maybe schools do not need to initiate an actual course: Bedside Manners 101, but some attention should be paid to getting physicians to understand the human side of patients' needs— their frailties, hopes, and yes, even despair. There is a lot out there in the world of medical practice which medical students never anticipate and can't comprehend, but it seldom is technical in nature. Medical schools do an excellent job on the tissue, bones, and muscles, on illnesses and technique. On the human and judgmental side, much room for improvement exists. Some physicians never gain these insights on their own. They just become too busy reading charts—including the Dow Jones—to concern themselves with their patients' feelings.

Medical technology in itself is for the most part marvelous. Nothing relieves a physician more or gives greater joy than when an advance in one's speciality allows for more effective treatment of an ailment. But human beings are complex creatures, and technology cannot do it on its own. The patient must always be more important than the disease. My superiors in their conference room treated blood cells; I watched a neat kid die.

Chapter VI

USING TECHNOLOGY WISELY

Let us now turn to the issue of the economics of medical technology. Questions of how technology is used, who pays the costs, and who receives the benefits are very complex and difficult ones. Yet a disturbing trend in medicine has developed, namely that 60-70 percent of all health care dollars are being spent on only 10 percent of individuals who receive medical care. This pattern of the allocation of resources is obviously troubling for a very simple reason: it suggests that expensive procedures may be available only to a portion of the public at large, yet the burden of funding medical and hospital expenses, and the insurance policies and government programs which underwrite them, are probably more evenly distributed. Ideally, the function of a democratic society is to create equal access to the law, and the majority of us share a belief that there should also be some sort of parity or equity in access to health care. The development of the advanced technology has created several ethical problems: 1) when should expensive or radical procedures be used, and 2) who will have, and who will be denied access to these expensive procedures, especially if they are too expensive to allocate to the entire population?

Part of the problem regarding the expense of radical procedures is that we often pass on the financing of them to the government or insurance companies. When someone is dying and is placed on a respirator and fed intravenously, most families will tell the doctor to "do anything needed to keep our loved one alive," knowing that the expensive cost will be covered by Medicare or the insurance company. Often oblivious to the quality of life of the dying individual, the family is relieved to know that death is being put off temporarily. I wonder, however, how many respirator plugs would be pulled *if* the family had to pay some share—say

25 percent—of the cost of all life sustaining radical procedures for the terminally ill. I have a very strong suspicion that even among those who actually had the resources, decisions would change. I do not mean to be crass or to suggest that most people do not truly care for their loved ones. I do mean to say that attitudes toward death, specifically a fear of it and a willingness to tolerate any condition so long as death is delayed, often cause resources to be tied up which could be put to more beneficial use. Again let me digress to my own experience.

When I was in medical school, the very first patient who was assigned to me, under the guidance of a physician of course, died within two hours. He had been brought into a hospital in a coma from a drug overdose. The standard clinical procedures, which we employed promptly and efficiently, were just not enough to revive the individual. The experience was very difficult for me. Young and idealistic, motivated to help my fellow man, my first patient was a cadaver within hours. I was depressed and almost immediately tried to develop a detachment from the situation, even though I had been eager to help a fellow human being. After only one patient, I was on the road to depersonalization and lack of involvement. Nobody in the medical school was prepared to help me—no course, no counselor, no advisor

94

was specifically assigned to helping the young would-be physician learn to cope with death and the loss of a patient. I had to eventually work out my feelings on my own, which I have done quite successfully, but it took much personal self-evaluation and self-education.

I would argue that many doctors in the profession and many people in our culture have unresolved feelings regarding death. Physicians tend to think of death in the same way I looked at it for that first patient—as a defeat, as losing a battle. A physician can only justify his performance if a body is still alive, quite apart from the condition it is in. How often then is life maintained with elaborate technical supports when in the normal course of events life would have already ceased, and for good and merciful reasons?

I firmly believe that physicians need to divest themselves of the idea that death is losing. It is not; it is an inevitable part of life and, as such, cannot be avoided. The finest doctor is not the one who puts death off at all costs, oblivious to all suffering and future promise of health; the finest doctor is one who attends death without fear and embarrassment, especially when the family or the dying individual needs the security of the physician—as in making the patient comfortable. It is possible to die with grace and love, and good physicians will attend on death without experiencing emotional trauma themselves.

Some would argue that my position is wrong, that life must be maintained at all costs because some new technological discovery may restore health. And I ask: even for an octogenarian whose body has been wracked with pain and for whom the debilitation of the disease has slowly destroyed the functioning of the body's organs? Yet how often do we see such lives sustained beyond the point of human endurance just because we as physicians do not wish to admit "defeat," or because some family member cannot accept the loss of a loved one? Physicians often know more than they say about what the prospects for future health are. When a patient has no chance for meaningful recovery, the physician at least owes the family an honest explanation and a forthright discussion regarding what the future options are, one of which should be to discuss how a patient can die with dignity. At times physicians tend to hide behind the technology without helping a family face the inevitable. The doctors who treated my young friend for leukemia are an example.

Questions of medical ethics and the use of technology are complex—almost impossible to discuss as generalizations because each individual case is unique. But some of the problems and expenses associated with technology could be alleviated were physicians and the general public more concerned with the quality of life and a little less averse to dealing with death directly and honestly. In the broadest sense, the principle which should apply is a question of the quality of life which the technology promises. For anyone, of whatever age, expensive diagnostic tools should be used if they promise to help identify how the patient might be able to sustain a meaningful existence. The decision should also be tilted in favor of the expense and the effort if a procedure offers any reasonable hope of meaningful life. But until we come to accept death and its inevitability, and until we as a profession are honest about what artificial life extension means both in suffering to patients and in falsified expectations, many resources will be wasted and used less effectively than they might be otherwise. The whole question is, incidentally, another one which should be broached in medical school—but generally isn't.

Another problem which is built into the present system of allopathic or mainstream medical care—and we often receive criticism for it from other health care practitioners—is that the medical profession benefits financially from disease. In fact, we tend to see individuals only when they are sick, only when they are "patients" eager to be relieved of pain and suffering. Obviously, it would be better were we able to place greater emphasis on and derive satisfaction from keeping people well. We might benefit from the logic of ancient Chinese medical practice, in which the physician was paid only when patients were healthy, but not when they were sick. While I do not recommend this as a course of action, it serves as a valuable insight. It is always more satisfying for me to find and head off a potential cancer than it is to treat one which has gone beyond a point at which it can be easily treated. The medical profession as a whole could be doing more to promote the concept of wellness.

Doctors also face monetary temptations because of the new technology. Lasers, for example, are exceptionally useful in treating a detached retina or for eliminating strawberry birth marks. But lasers are not necessary for many procedures they are commonly used for. Warts, for example, can be removed for $50 with a trusty old electro-desiccator like the one which hangs on my wall. Laser devices cost $30,000-40,000. Doctors who have purchased them must receive a return on the investment. So they commonly advertise their ability to do "laser surgery" and charge $600 for the removal of the warts, with the exact same result as the $50 procedure. Once the expensive device is paid for, the technology can be used as an excuse to demand large fees and thus higher salaries.

The media attention given to radical medical technologies also creates a problem for practicing physicians. The public at large comes to believe that virtually any disease can be cured and that physicians should have easy remedies in their black bags for all ailments. Ironically, the realization that radical procedures exist is liable to encourage irresponsibility in the living habits of the general populace because of a mistaken belief that virtually any problem can be cured via a medication or surgical procedure. The truth is, advances in medicine are not made evenly across the board. Certain illnesses still pose intractable problems. While noteworthy advances have been made in recent years in understanding diseases like cancer, the practical advantages of the insights and the development of effective modes of treatment for at least some forms of cancer may yet be some years in the future.

The tendency to assume that doctors know everything and can cure any malady also leads to much patient grumbling and dissatisfaction when easy cures are not forthcoming—an issue that probably contributes to at least some malpractice suits. Patients will sometimes beome angry with physicians who warn that a diagnosis may not be exact or a test may not prove conclusively whether a particular disease is responsible for the patient's problems. Or patients will be dissatisfied when a physician cannot make a diagnosis based on some rather vague description of symptoms or without ordering expensive tests. All these problems point to a need for physicians to take time with and educate their patients, not merely turn them loose with medications which, when misused, are themselves liable to cause further problems.

No matter what treatments or technology is applied, human beings will still be mortal. If technology is too often used in an attempt to deny mortality, competition will become fierce for the limited resources. But whatever we do with technology, we will best be able to afford it and we will best serve the public if we treat patients as humans, using the technology when it benefits the patient, and not as a detached substitute for personal care.

Section IV

MALPRACTICE

To change the (legal) system will be difficult . . . but it's not impossible. It is important to work for such a change. If we fail, access to quality health care will continue to diminish for the American people.

Ulrich Danckers, M.D.
President, Chicago Medical Society
Chicago Medicine Magazine
October 21, 1989

Salus Populi suprema est lex. (The good of the people is the chief law.)

Cicero
De Legibus

Chapter VII

THE HIDDEN THREAT

Physicians and health care professionals point to the malpractice crisis as the greatest problem facing American medicine today. Lawsuits brought against physicians and hospitals lead to increases in fees which, in turn, force insurance companies to raise their premiums for health insurance to levels that become prohibitively expensive for many Americans. When tens of millions of Americans cannot afford medical insurance, many fail to receive adequate treatment, and the cost of paying for those who are being treated must be picked up by the public sector. In certain high risk specialities, physicians are at the point at which no matter what they charge for their services, they cannot realize a profit because of insurance premiums which can exceed one hundred thousand dollars per year. These monetary pressures cause the cost of medical care to grow at a much greater rate than inflation. The public grumbles about the increased expense, but the situation does not improve. The present adversarial atmosphere shows no signs of abating.

Before we consider the legal side of this issue, I would first point out the ugly underside of the problem—the part most Americans are probably not aware of—namely that the malpractice crisis has had a terribly negative effect on the actual practice of medicine. Physicians, being human and therefore naturally inclined to protect themselves from external threats, now often practice medicine less than optimally because the malpractice crisis dictates that they "protect themselves at all costs" rather than put the patient's own best interest first. Decisions about how to care for a patient are often dictated by the physician's expectations of what a lawyer would look for in the event a problem arose in treatment. Needless to say, such fears can interfere with the physician's method of practicing medicine. Because of this fear, an increasing number of X-rays, laboratory tests, and unnecessary follow up visits are scheduled by doctors. The cost is borne by the patients via increased fees. Even if a physician were inclined to exercise independent judgment on behalf of a patient, the hospitals in which they work are liable to create policies which will force doctors to follow procedures intended to avoid a lawsuit at all costs.

Emergency rooms serve as a typical first example. Nowadays anyone brought into an emergency room in a crisis situation may be subjected to X-rays and other tests which at one time would not have been ordered and are normally not necessary. The procedures are required just to make sure that the doctor does not do anything to the patient which some judge or jury at some later date might consider inappropriate. It does not take much imagination to realize the consequences of requiring tests of questionable value in emergency situations.

In spite of federal laws, emergency rooms at some hospitals have turned away patients because of established policies designed to protect the hospital from undesirable lawsuits. Some hospitals, for example, will not treat rape victims unless they have been injured by the rapist— shot, stabbed, or beaten—in addition to being raped. In a recent case, a woman claims she was turned away from a hospital because of such a policy—allegedly one of three rape victims turned away in one night. She is now suing the hospital. The purpose and function of a hospital should be to help people in need. But the hospitals in question turn away rape victims because "of the liability," and because doctors may become involved in legal issues associated with a crime. Failing in the role of helping the victim because of policies which are intended to protect the hospital from lawsuits, the hospital administration finds itself faced with a suit anyway. In this case, an attitude of mutual distrust and monetary competition now separates hospital and patient.

Lawsuits are also creating a crisis of service, especially in so-called high risk areas like obstetrics. Not only have many general practitioners been driven out of the field because of increased malpractice premiums, but so have obstetricians themselves. Because a baby can experience various forms of trauma during birth and subsequently suffer irreversible damage, the practice of delivering babies becomes, by definition, high risk. That the risks result from natural causes which have existed throughout all human history does not lessen the threat of lawsuits. In fact, many birth defects are the result, not of any physician's actions, but of problems in the development of a fetus. At times—though certainly not in all cases—the problems can arise because women do not follow their doctor's advice and warnings during the pre-natal period. They smoke or drink or use recreational drugs when pregnant. Other problems are genetic and beyond anyone's control. A damaged infant, however, can produce a huge settlement from a jury. Our society and our court system do not allow for acts of God in medical care. By definition, the physician or hospital is assigned the blame. Juries are very sensitive to permanent, irreversible damage to any infant, and it is not always easy to prove to a jury that the physician in charge was not the cause of the child's defect. These problems have led to a large increase in the number of Caesarean sections, which are more expensive than natural childbirth, require a longer period of recuperation, and can pose greater risks to the mother. At times, the option is necessary, but far too often the procedure is being used to head off potential lawsuits. For the most part, modern medical techniques are responsible for very safe births, but since the very process of giving birth is high risk, the malpractice premiums for anyone who delivers babies are enough to drive conscientious physicians away from the service.

While as a practicing dermatologist, I am not generally in the forefront of the malpractice crisis, nevertheless, I am aware of its impact on my own practice. Because of threats of possible lawsuits, I will not write a prescription for the best anti-acne drug on the market today *if* the patient is a female of child bearing age. While acne may seem like a frivolous problem to some, severe cases of acne can cause such a crisis of self-identity that patients occasionally show suicidal tendencies when relief from the condition is not found. The drug Accutane has proven very successful in clearing up extremely bad cases of acne, but it also carries with it a small, but real, potential for adversely affecting a fetus. My own personal preference would be to administer the drug to women of child bearing age after clear counseling and an explanation of the risks involved. The woman who uses it should not be sexually active or should be certain to avoid conception. In the present atmosphere, however, not even a signed release is certain to hold up in court, and so I am often forced to use drugs which are less effective and have potentially greater side effects—even when I know that a woman could be better served by the use of the preferred drug. Not even a company sponsored program which promotes contraception awareness has swayed me from my decision to avoid the drug in young women of child bearing age.

Everywhere in the medical profession, doctors have their own tales of how they have altered their practices to protect themselves from lawsuits. In virtually every case, the patient is not served as well as he or she otherwise might have been. In fact, the whole process of being sued has had a terrible impact on the lives of many physicians, especially young ones. I recently had an opportunity to talk with a young physician who had just received his first notification of a malpractice suit. Only two years in practice, the physician has an excellent reputation and a bright future. He admitted to me that the threat of the suit had seriously disrupted his life. When I discussed the case with him, it was apparent that he was not at fault. A patient had had a drug reaction which fell within the defined possibilities of the drug being used. He expeditiously treated the patient and advised a course of action to minimize the problem. Nevertheless, he is being sued. Being fairly new in the profession, he fears that his entire practice and future may be ruined. Because of his anxiety, his home life is being disrupted and his relationship to patients is being threatened. He frankly admits that every time he sees a patient, he now sees a potential enemy. That is simply tragic, given his impeccable character and reputation and his honest commitment to the highest standards of the profession. Even if he wins the suit, which I expect he will, is he to become another physician who will depersonalize his practice, or who will develop calloused feelings to patients he is trying to help?

The type of fear which has been instilled in doctors also has adverse effects on patients. Many doctors I have spoken with now routinely

109

advise their patients of worst case possibilities when diagnosing them, not because there is a high probability that the patient will succumb to or be debilitated by a disease, but as a way of lowering expectations so that the doctor is not blamed for the effects of the disease. The danger with such an approach is that such predictions can become self-fulfilling prophecies. If an expert tells you that you are very sick and you have little chance of recovering, the anxiety and defeatist attitude you develop may weaken your resolve and will to fight the disease. I find this tactic inhumane and counter-productive although I can understand why doctors who treat high risk patients feel compelled to protect themselves.

The malpractice crisis is one that must be addressed soon and aggressively. Before I move on to concrete recommendations in the next chapter, I would like to touch on one more peripheral issue of malpractice, mainly because it is so closely tied in to the human side of the practice of medicine. The issue is one of the propriety of physician-patient contact.

Much attention is given in our culture to issues of sex: the advertising of an amazing array of products is predicated on their ability to enhance sex appeal; movies and television programs seem obsessed with treating interpersonal relationships as questions of sexual identity. In spite of the wholesale marketing of sex which, if nothing else, represents a publicly honest statement of the significance of the role of sex in our lives, the public at large seems to be terribly frightened regarding issues of sex, perhaps because of the attention sexual crimes receive in the media. Cases of child molestation gain national attention and lead to rigid reactions against the public display of affection of any kind, especially for professionals who treat the public at large. If a teacher at a pre-school hugs a child, he or she runs a risk of having that behavior misunderstood or misinterpreted. And so it is in the medical profession. While I would be the first to admit that physicians need to have the greatest respect for the privacy and dignity of their patients—everyone is aware of the embarrassment of disrobing in front of a stranger to say nothing of being examined and probed—I fear that the threat of malpractice in the form of claims of sexual advances is causing physicians never to touch their patients in any way without a medical instrument in their hands. This, I think, is nonsense.

I have heard many stories from patients who have spoken of the value of a physician's touch, but I would like to relate one at length because it ties in with a number of issues of doctor-patient relationships. I have a good friend who once ingested, quite by accident of course, several parasites and became quite ill. The resultant diarrhea caused him to lose fifteen pounds in a week, and he went to see a physician. Since no external examination or general history could identify the problem, the doctor prescribed an anti-diarrhea medication and sent my friend home to see if his problem would clear up, specifically warning him that if the medication did not help, further examination and some testing would certainly be necessary. The young man tried the medication but, instead of being relieved, began vomiting. The next day he returned to the doctor's office where, because of his condition, a sensitive nurse immediately escorted him to an examination room so he could lie down. When the physician entered, he took one look at my friend's pallid face and shivering body, gently touched him on the side of the head, and said, "Son, we're going to put you in the hospital until we figure out what is wrong and make you well again."

As my friend says, "I can't tell you how much that touch meant. He had obviously seen with one look what bad shape I was in, and he wanted to convey his concern. But his words alone couldn't have done it; it was his touch, his attitude and demeanor which gave me confidence in him. Though I had never gone to him before this problem, I was sure he was a professional—and he was. A week after I got out of the hospital, just when I was back to my normal self and feeling I could eat anything—well, I got sick again. Boy was I depressed. But two minutes later I received a phone call from the doctor. 'We found another parasite, and I have to issue another medication or else you'll be back where you started.' The call wasn't a coincidence. The man was thorough. He did not take my seeming quick recovery at the hospital at face value. He had ordered complete follow up tests and discovered a second type of parasite. But it all came down to that touch and the tone of his voice—I had confidence that he cared and he knew medicine.''

Incidentally, some patients might have sued the physician. The first medication he administered, after all, produced an adverse reaction for this particular patient in this particular situation. But the physician was following intelligent practice. When a patient shows up in a doctor's office with a condition which cannot be diagnosed accurately without elaborate, expensive, and time consuming tests, physicians often take a cautious approach: since the overwhelming percentage of such problems will clear up by themselves, the physician seeks to relieve the symptoms and waits to see if the condition improves. Normally, such problems are the result of a stomach virus or of having eaten some bacterially contaminated food. When the problem did not clear up, the doctor acted at once and ordered tests which identified the problem. Once the parasites were identified, several excellent medications eliminated them without side effects. The doctor took a prudent and wise course of action. Nowadays, he might be forced to undertake expensive tests immediately, out of a fear that a patient might be an opportunist.

In my own practice, I quite commonly touch my patients, not merely during the necessary contact of a diagnosis, but to demonstrate the closeness of our medical, yet human, relationship. I am happily married and have no need to seek any sexual gratification from such contact. But when at the end of a diagnosis, a patient may be greatly relieved and wishes to give a hug of joy, or deeply disturbed and threatened and seeks some solace in a hug against the fear, I am not going to hold back just because someone else is perverse. I am no threat and I am pleased if patients can sense my concern for them and show emotion, whether of relief or distress. Obviously, tact is required. The external demeanor of the patient and the length of our working relationship may dictate what contact is made. But even a reassuring touch of one hand upon another helps show the patient that there is a closeness and concern which represents my determination to do my best for the individual.

The sex that is used to sell products in the mass media is often perverse because it *is* pornographic—by which I mean, it is at once depersonalized and erotic. The contact I make with a patient is neither, and I am not going to stop doing something which can benefit the human spirit just because someone else is perverted. The whole defensiveness regarding touch is absurd; after all, psychologists tell us that people who have sexual problems are often those who have been deprived of affection expressed through touching and physical contact.

Chapter VIII

THE LEGAL ANGLE

As I discuss the legal aspects of the malpractice crisis, let me begin by establishing my premise. Malpractice does exist and is a real problem, and the role of the legal profession in identifying and exposing negligence can be beneficial. On the other hand, after paying attention for years to the type of suits which have been filed and litigated, I can say without reservation that the overwhelming majority of medical malpractice suits have little merit or are downright frivolous.

If the majority of suits lack merit, why—the reader might ask—do they continue to be filed? One would suppose that trial judges and juries would be fed up with hearing nonsense

116

malpracice cases and would see the lack of substance in the majority of them. One of the answers to the question is that most cases never go to trial. Because the cost of defending a physician in front of a judge and jury is so expensive, insurance companies quite commonly seek settlements outside of court, even when a suit has no real merit. This willingness to capitulate for the sake of keeping costs down actually contributes to an increasing number of suits. Then too, when cases are brought before juries, decisions are often reached based on how well attorneys can elicit a response from a jury. Individuals on a jury do not have medical training and they are liable to be influenced by emotional issues, as for example the problems and expenses a family will face when raising a child who was permanently injured during childbirth. Since malpractice cases are civil suits in which the "preponderance of evidence" can be considered sufficient to render a verdict—unlike criminal suits wherein the defendant is presumed innocent until proven guilty—it is easy for jury members to assume that, since doctors and insurance companies have deep pockets, they ought to provide support for a child who was harmed at birth.

My own first experience in malpractice occurred during a post graduate year of training in pediatrics when I was part of a team which treated a baby born with multiple physical defects. Everyone involved with the patient or whose name appeared on the chart for any reason was named in the malpractice suit. This practice of naming a large number of defendants, incidentally, has now become a standard procedure. Besides the obvious legal reason—an attorney not wishing to let anyone with any responsibility escape the suit—I strongly suspect that this tactic is used as a form of leverage to force out-of-court settlements. The more complicated the suit, the harder and the more expensive it is to defend.

I did not receive a subpoena in the case until a few years later during my dermatology residency. Needless to say, I was shocked because I had very specific recollections of the effort which the physician in charge had given to the infant. To this day, I have never seen a patient handled with greater commitment. We moved with inordinate speed in an attempt to care for the child. The child was born in a hospital which was incapable of handling his problems and, of necessity, the infant was transferred to our hospital's high risk nursery. Usually we would wait for an ambulance to take us to the location of the infant in trouble. But because we were told about the difficult problems, the head of the Neonatal Intensive Care Unit took the team in a private car to save precious minutes. In the course of saving and sustaining the child's life, unavoidable problems and complications arose. But the problems existed before the physician I was working under ever saw the infant.

Faced with the task of raising a retarded child, the parents blamed the physician and hospital and filed a lawsuit. Reading the entire complaint made me feel sick to my stomach. In twenty pages or so, our staff was personally accused of what sounded to me like intentional crimes against humanity. Indictments from the Nuremberg tribunals probably used more gentle language. I felt threatened, scared, and filled with a terrible sense of anguish. Who could have dreamed up such allegations? Did the attorney and family really believe that we wanted to hurt the child? All the doctors involved, myself included, had done our very best in very difficult circumstances, but attorneys were now making public statements that we were incompetent and that we had destroyed the life of a child. The moment was unbelievably painful. One of my first reactions was to think that had we been less efficient, the child would certainly have died and the suit would never have been initiated. My feelings demonstrate how easily a physician can become calloused when professional commitment and competence are interpreted as reckless behavior. The day I received the complaint, I was so paralyzed with mixed emotions that I

119

could not perform my duties in the clinic. I went home to share my emotions with my wife and family.

This sort of shock is a common response of doctors to their first lawsuit. My father-in-law helped ease much of the pain by getting me to see that, since I knew I was not to blame for the problems, I need not be disturbed by the accusations. I awakened quickly to the realization that malpractice suits would be part of the cost of practicing medicine. Sooner or later, I realized, considering the state of our society, every practicing physician might have to face such charges, even if they were groundless.

Because of the suit, I was required to attend a deposition for the purpose of collecting information about the case. The deposition was an all day affair during which the plaintiff's attorney attempted to wear me down with questions he knew I could not answer. He must have believed that he could badger me into making some mistake which would make his case for him. He was very disappointed.

Nevertheless, for me, the interrogation was an exercise in fear, frustration, and anger. The attorney displayed at least twenty X-rays from a stack of perhaps one hundred, asking a myriad of questions about each. What did I think about this particular X-ray? Could I interpret the X-ray for him? What was my opinion with regard to the course of action which should have been followed because of what the X-ray showed? My firm but polite answer to each question was identical: that not being a radiologist or a pediatrician, I had no opinion about the film. I had not interpreted the X-rays during the course of treatment and I saw no need to do so now.

The interrogation was a frightening experience for me, but as I attempted to understand what happened, I confronted at least one of the contributing factors in the malpractice crisis: the mutual lack of understanding between physicians and attorneys. Doctors have little experience with the adversary/advocate nature of the legal profession. Attorneys are only doing the job for which they were trained, namely to be advocates for their clients in a system based on adversary relationship. Attorneys pit their skills against each other in a battle of proving their client right and the other attorney's client wrong. The real practice of law involves lawyers trying to get as much for their client as possible without regard to justice or fairness.

I once asked an attorney how he could possibly defend a criminal who he knew had committed the crime of which he stood accused. Each man, he suggested, is due his day in court, and it is the responsibility of the attorney to make sure the state proves its case against his client. Otherwise, as in a dictatorship, anyone could be imprisoned and punished based on falsified information.

My friend's comments express the noble and lofty purpose of the law. Reality is often different from theory. Instead of seeking justice, many attorneys use technicalities in the language of the law to allow guilty parties to get off without any penalty.

Physicians do not understand the legal system. It is an alien world to us. Our training places us in a different competition: against pain, disease, and suffering. As business oriented as we might become, we have never been trained to fight against another human but to struggle as an advocate for humans against a non-human foe.

Thus, what is business as usual for attorneys leaves us wounded and confused. Attorneys who compete in a case are able to sit down to a friendly dinner after the judgment is rendered, no matter who wins or loses. Defending or representing their clients is what they do to earn money. They do not understand the sensitive feelings doctors have regarding patients. Therefore, attorneys probably do not understand the emotional burden a malpractice suit creates for physicians. My own experience tells me that not even those attorneys who defend doctors against malpractice suits realize what a shock it is for physicians to be told that they were not doing their best or that they are incompetent. To attorneys, the matter becomes one of manipulating arguments, and doctors are grossly offended when lawyers who know little about medicine bastardize the practice of medicine with legalistic terminology.

This adversarial nature of the legal profession is something which I have come to understand although the awareness does not really ease the feeling of threat when any physician is grilled either at a deposition or on the jury stand. In rape cases, for example, the defendant's attorney is liable to try to make a fool out of a physician for the failure to follow "proper procedures" in taking and recording hair and semen samples. A sensitive doctor who was simply doing his job without anticipating being questioned about it in public by a skilled interrogator is liable to have to face tricky and difficult questions, quite unprepared for the grilling. Then doctors, of course, become reluctant to provide services if the legalistic concerns take precedence over treating or helping the patient. The result is another one of those horrible problems which arises out of the present system: doctors appearing to be insensitive to rape. But they are motivated by fear—fear of attorneys and depositions. And the fear is almost always a problem of a lack of communication and understanding.

If this text does nothing else, I hope it will promote some understanding of this massive failure of communication between two professions. If citizens are outraged by physicians who seem reluctant to treat rape cases, they should at least know that the problem usually arises because some honest and caring doctor was publicly disparaged and smeared on a witness stand, not for actual incompetence, but for not having anticipated legalistic badgering intended to get a rapist off the hook.

The first malpractice case I was involved in was eventually settled out of court though I only found out about the settlement quite by accident when phoning one of the other doctors who was named in the suit. I was relieved not to be required to spend days in court away from my newly opened practice of dermatology, but I was also stunned that a case in which I was accused of behavior suitable to a horror movie was settled without my knowledge or consent.

Throughout the country, hospital hallways are filled with stories of physicians sued for minimal reasons. The first suit in which I was specifically identified as a culprit does not even merit serious consideration in the discussion of malpractice. But it is an example of the type of suit commonly being filed against physicians and so I will offer some specifics. It is valuable to keep in mind as you read the details of this case that, even though the case was thrown out as lacking merit, I had to spend a great deal of time and expense in preparing to defend myself against the claim.

A few years ago, I treated a young man who had multiple genital warts, which are highly contagious and could easily have spread to his wife. If only a few warts had been present, I would have used the most common procedure, surgical removal, an inexpensive and relatively painless process. But this young man had hundreds of growths. Surgery was impossible. So I prescribed a topical cream which provokes a local irritation. The resulting inflammation causes white blood cells to enter the area, a process which is designed to help the body "discover" the virus responsible for the warts so that the body's immune system will destroy it. If applied to the groin away from the genitals, the cream will cause mild irritation. But if used directly on a man's sex organs, sensitive tissue can become swollen, with rather painful results. To avoid problems, I routinely instruct patients in the proper method of using the cream and in the theory of what will happen to clear up the problem. This man received the full explanation.

He did not follow my instructions and he applied the medication to both his penis and scrotum. The result was a painful irritation which became mildly infected in response to his scratching the area. The basis of the suit was a lack of consortium. The patient claimed that he and his wife could not have sex during the week he was irritated by the medication. For seven loveless days, he asked for compensation of $150,000, in spite of the fact that his problem resulted from a complete failure to follow specific instructions given both by the physician and on the medication's packaging. He experienced no residual or permanent damage to any part of his body. Now, I fully concede that at times sex can be priceless, both literally and metaphorically, but $21,000 a night is frankly a rip-off.

It is easy for me to joke about such an issue now, but what is not funny is that a lawyer helped this patient file his complaint. Malpractice, in fact, is seldom humorous; it creates much trauma for physicians, most of it unjustifiable. And we commonly feel as if the plaintiffs are attempting to make a quick killing.

Before I begin to suggest possible reforms and ways of lessening the malpractice crisis, I think it will be worthwhile to make several points about the practice of medicine. Virtually any procedure in medicine entails some risk, and no drug or medication is completely safe for every patient in every situation. If physicians are to be blamed for everything bad which happens to patients who are ill, we might as well close shop and go home. Every drug on the market has the potential for having an adverse effect on someone. Even when physicians assure patients that a particular drug is safe, the product descriptions will include explanations which show that in rare cases, problems can arise. If only one in ten thousand patients will experience an adverse reaction, some physician somewhere is liable to be blamed for the problem. When a patient seeks help from a physician, he or she must realize that some risk is entailed in any procedure or regimen. Frankly, modern medical procedures and medications are forever being refined so that the problems associated with them generally grow smaller and smaller, but risk can never reach absolute zero. Nor can the physician take total responsibility for everything that happens to a patient.

Doctors cannot do their jobs if their hands are tied by a system which blames them for everything. While I do not have the space in this book to discuss what constitutes professional negligence or incompetence in a variety of fields of medicine, it seems to me that physicians should lose malpractice suits only if it can be demonstrated that they were truly negligent and that the steps they took were at variance with reasonable and prudent medical practice. The most common logical fallacy which plagues human thinking is the *post hoc* fallacy, the assumption that because one condition follows another in time, the first must be the cause of the second. When patients experience a problem, it is common to blame the physician or hospital for it, even though neither may have caused the problem. But cause-effect relationships relating to health can easily be misunderstood or misinterpreted. Given the fact that it is a natural human tendency to want to blame someone else for problems—watch any two siblings explain to their parents who was to blame for a fight—doctors and hospitals find themselves blamed for many problems for which they are not responsible.

As we search for ways to lessen the impact of the malpractice crisis, suggested solutions should guarantee that the legal process is not destroyed. Some cases may be open to argument, even were experienced physicians to serve as the jury. Justice requires that the process of argument remain free. Yet at the same time, the system must be reformed so that it cannot easily be abused and manipulated to the advantage of those who merely seek to reap profit from it. One of the real tragedies of the present crisis is that when real malpractice occurs and a person who has been victimized and lost a capacity should be compensated for the malpractice, the individual will probably be forced to wait many long years before the case can even be heard because the courts are tied up with so many suits of questionable merit. Those who deserve justice, in other words, cannot get it and may be forced to settle for a small monetary compensation which will not cover their expenses and losses.

One possible way of reducing lawsuits and the cost to everyone concerned is to require, by law, that before a medical malpractice lawsuit is filed, the plaintiff and the physician meet with a third, neutral party to discuss the problems which allegedly arose. If my premise is correct, namely that the majority of cases are not the result of real malpractice, such meetings with an ombudsman could be of great benefit in resolving conflict and would even have an additional benefit of improving the practice of medicine.

Let us assume in one case that the contention of malpractice arose because the physician, while not actually being incompetent, rushed a patient or failed to communicate well. The arbitration might serve as an eye opener in letting a physician understand how and why patients are offended and why they feel that the burden of their problems should be borne by the physician. Were the physician to understand the cause of the patient's anger or problem, the problem might be resolved in any number of ways without costly litigation. The physician might apologize and, at times, might even offer to make amends for perceived wrongdoing. If such an ombudsman system existed, it might help reduce the burden on the present overloaded legal system, but more importantly, doctors who now complain of malpractice suits in the isolation of their medical offices would be able to confront the complaints directly and might learn what is bothering patients and how to better satisfy their patients in the future.

Let us now assume that in other specific cases, the doctor was not at fault at all, but the patient honestly feels that a physician did something seriously wrong. Why might such a situation arise? For a variety of reasons. The patient may not be well educated about medicine, or the patient may be venting anger against authority figures. Since doctors are traditionally looked upon as authority or parent figures, some patients vent their unresolved anger toward authority by attacking doctors. Another possibility is that patients are attempting to assuage their own guilt. Parents, for example, when faced with a newborn who has been damaged, often direct their anger and frustration at a physician. Along with the anger comes an even more destructive emotion—guilt. Someone must be responsible for what happened. The feelings of guilt can be overwhelming for parents. It is not human nature to easily accept blame for a circumstance. Since you can't blame Mother Nature, an abstract concept, the physician often becomes the target of the anger.

How then could such a system benefit the patient? The patient, too, might be educated by the process, by realizing that doctors cannot be held responsible for every problem associated with a disease. A person who is suffering from one illness, for example, may be weakened to the point that a second affliction will strike the body. The physician certainly does not introduce additional disease and cannot always deal with multiple infections easily because the treatment of one may produce complications with the other.

Such meetings might also serve to educate patients who are responsible for their own poor results, either because they fail to follow instructions or do not take medications. Many patients do not take responsibility for their follow-up care. An ombudsman might be able to help patients understand their role in maintaining and promoting health.

Obviously individuals who act as ombudsmen should know quite a bit about medicine and law, in addition to psychology. Training for the position might entail much education, but were such a system to develop, it could be beneficial not merely in settling grievances, but in making both physicians and patients sensitive to each other's needs and problems.

Now obviously an ombudsman system would not clear up all cases. All patients would not be satisfied, even when their cases were weak or

131

frivolous, and some real malpractice suits would have to be litigated. Nevertheless, if the system were to reduce the number of suits initiated, it would benefit the overburdened legal system immensely, partly by allowing the remaining suits to be litigated more expeditiously. Furthermore, if the majority of complaints could be resolved, insurance companies would not be quite so willing to settle matters out of court just because a plaintiff hired a high powered attorney. This might allow the insurance companies to concentrate their resources and defend doctors who are unquestionably in the right. The impact of winning a large number of cases would be to discourage the filing of complaints of little or no merit.

I would also recommend that judges be given the authority to make plaintiffs pay the defendants' legal fees *if* a suit is deemed to be frivolous. Had the suit regarding the genital warts been brought to trial, for example, I see no reason why I or my insurance company should have to pay for the legal expenses to defend me. If someone from the public wants to play a lottery by taking a chance and suing a physician, he or she must at least have some reasonable grounds for the basis of the suit. The individual's right to sue must be defended, but plaintiffs should realize that if they are just out to take advantage of the system, they must entail a risk.

If you want to play in a lottery, you at least have to pay the price of the ticket. When the system exacts some price, then plaintiffs will sue only when they are convinced that malpractice existed, not just to make a fast buck.

Which leads me to another problem of the present American system as it applies to malpractice. Most malpractice suits are taken by lawyers without requiring that the plaintiff pay any fees to the attorney. Many lawyers simply indicate to their clients that they will take a case on a contingency fee basis. In effect, they say, "You don't have to pay me a dime. I'll take my fee from the settlement, whether judicial or out-of-court." Obviously, such a system can and is easily abused. For example, an attorney will almost immediately ask for twice the amount of money which the offended party thinks they are entitled to since attorneys usually take half of the settlement as their reward. This radically inflates the cost of medical insurance to everyone for a simple reason: even when a malpractice case is successfully litigated and the patient deserves compensation, the cost to the insurer and, thus, to everyone who uses medical services increases because the settlement subsidizes lawyers at rates far exceeding their normal fees.

In Great Britain at the present time, the contingency fee system is outlawed. American trial lawyers would like to see the ground rules changed in England. But after looking at the abuses of malpractice, I feel it would be wiser were we to eliminate or greatly reduce the contingency fee system in this country. Right now attorneys are motivated to attack, attack, attack, based on the premise that even if they win only a small percentage of malpractice cases, they will make considerable money due to the inordinately large settlements.

American trial lawyers say the poor would not have representation were there no contingency fee system. But that is not true for a number of reasons. First of all, lawyers could still be paid out of a settlement were they paid for the actual work they did rather than half of a massive amount, which a jury probably assumes is actually being awarded to compensate the victim of the malpractice. Then too, lawyers can and should be willing to do a certain amount of work *pro bono*. If an injured party had a good case, lawyers who were motivated to help an injured party would certainly take the case.

Another reform which would be helpful would be to make successfully litigated malpractice suits offer compensation commensurate with damage. In workmen's compensation suits, the loss of various bodily parts are assigned a specific value, as is the loss of life. In medical malpractice there is no such standard; recompense for pain and suffering often exceeds by many times the amount of money which is ever needed to compensate for the loss of capacity. If a physician makes a gross mistake and causes a person serious damage, that physician should be responsible for making the person whole. In so far as he cannot, he owes compensation; in most cases, this can be done only via monetary award. Let us assume that a person has been made a quadriplegic by a physician's error. The victim is certainly owed lost salary, the retrofitting of a house, and the purchase price of a specialized vehicle which can transport him. The compensation should undoubtedly cover these expensive items. If a physician is responsible, he and his insurance company should have to answer for such expenses. But if all those items are covered by, for instance, one million dollars, which would guarantee that the individual's and his family's needs would be taken care of, then why should he be given ten million, and the attorney an additional ten million? In some cases of which I am aware, families which have won settlements for a child's birth defects have used the moneys not to guarantee the future well-being of the child, but to live a high rolling life style. Perhaps we need court appointed administrators to ensure that money is not sidetracked, especially when settlements are made on behalf of children.

Another point which I think is important is that the compensatory fees which are due should guarantee the well-being of the person who was injured by the malpractice. The system should not produce a lottery wherein moneys awarded create a wealthy estate for the descendants of the injured party, and certainly not for the attorney's descendants to the seventh generation.

We need a strong legal system—it is our defense against totalitarianism. Everyone must have access to the courts. But at present, the malpractice system is perverted by materialism; the unnecessary lawsuits are to law what greed is to medicine.

Reforms, if they do come, will take time. In the meantime, I believe physicians can help alleviate the crisis if they do not let fear get in their way. Physicians who listen carefully to their patients, spend adequate amounts of time with them, and who take responsibility for own their mistakes have an extremely small number of lawsuits. Some people will sue anyone, and if a doctor comes across one of these patients, a suit may result. But we can greatly reduce the number of lawsuits and the cost of medical care in general by practicing medicine with a greater commitment to care than to money. This might mean seeing fewer patients and taking home less salary, but in the long run, the cost of a malpractice suit is much higher.

Choosing to practice as though lawyers were not enemies might sound crazy, but that has become the routine in my office. Each of my patients has my full time and attention. As much as possible, they are aware of everything to expect in the way of results and complications. Mistakes do happen, and I freely admit them and take responsibility for them. It is possible, after all, to make a mistake in a diagnosis. The human body is exceptionally complex, and many diseases closely mimic each other. When I do make a mistake, I do whatever is in my power to correct the mistake, and I do not charge for any correction which is made. Some of my patients have told me stories of other doctors who have made mistakes in their health care and then attempted to charge them additional fees to fix the mistakes. They found this unforgivable. Those physicians, by their actions, are playing with fire and inviting an angry patient to institute a lawsuit.

To me, part of the solution to the malpractice problem is simple. If we, as physicians, are attentive to our patients, and if we give away a fair share of free care, the public will redevelop their bond of love with the members of our profession. It is very hard to sue someone you love and admire, and in whom, during times of crisis, you place your trust.

Section V

SOLUTIONS

Historically, movements for social change have all operated in much the same way. A paternal leadership has convinced people of the need for change . . . telling them what to do and when to do it. The new social movements operate on a different assumption of human potential: the belief that individuals . . . can generate solutions from their own commitment and creativity.

Marilyn Ferguson,
The Aquarian Conspiracy

The 1990s represent an extremely important, even crucial, decade in the history of medicine. During this time, it is our opportunity, indeed our responsibility, to take steps necessary to deliver this beloved old learned profession of ours into the next millennium intact as a true profession— not merely as a trade or business.

George D. Lundberg, M.D.
JAMA, January 5, 1990

Chapter IX

THE FUTURE

Does the medical crisis referred to in the introduction of this book have a solution? You will excuse me for equivocating, but the answer is both yes and no. If we assume that solutions have to be dictated by governments, legislators, the American Medical Association, or any other organization, then the answer is no. If we have to wait for someone else to correct the problems, they will worsen before solutions are found. If on the other hand, each of us resolves to contribute to Making Medicine Work, then the problems will abate. No human system can be perfect, but I honestly believe that we can maintain and improve medical services when enough individuals place the quality of health care before all other considerations. For physicians this means putting the well-being of our patients before our salaries; for the public at large, this means working at promoting wellness. One of the most encouraging signs of future promise is that constructive changes are already taking place in every section of the country. We are constantly learning about physicians, health professionals, and lay volunteers who are using creative strategies to solve problems. And physicians who hear about our work are calling to find out how they can contribute. This concluding chapter will be dedicated to demonstrating how various individuals and organizations have "made medicine work" with creative solutions to problems in the medical health field.

MAKING MEDICINE WORK

Making Medicine Work is a non-profit foundation whose goal is to promote solutions to the problems which face the medical profession and to disseminate information on ways in which the general health of the population can be improved. It is absolutely essential that the reader understand the underlying philosophy of the foundation and how that philosophy can contribute to the promotion of health and wise medical practice. Our philosophy is based on an extension of the principles upon which this country was founded, principles which are sometimes referred to as "Jeffersonian democracy." What we envision is a society in which individuals take responsibility for their own health, and a system in which the physicians and other health care practitioners enroll the general populace in that effort. In recent years with the increase in marvelous technology, we have seen a tendency for patients to place doctors on a pedestal, to make them an "aristocracy" to whom the rest of the population turns to "undo their physical maladies." The patient "contributes" a disease, and the doctor is supposed to offer a technical solution to the problem. Such a system, however, has certain built in liabilities which have contributed to the crisis in medicine. When people do not work at being healthy and when they find that doctors cannot cure their every ailment, an adversarial relationship between doctor and patient develops; in many cases, lawsuits arise out of claims of malpractice. Costs rise, and health professionals, compensating for the threat of lost income, begin to compete with each other in attracting patients to their specialities. They take on more and more patients to maintain their income levels and lifestyles, and the quality of the service they offer erodes as work loads and stress increase. Patients, in turn, become suspicious of professionals.

One possible way of solving this problem is through government interference—via a system of socialized medicine. But, if the government were to run the entire health care system, the results would be horrendous. Certainly, we ought to have learned something from the recent collapse of planned economies all over eastern Europe. Centralized government control is not the answer.

The answer lies in individual initiative. At *Making Medicine Work*, we do not profess to have the answer to all problems regarding medicine. We do feel, however, that if medicine is to be effective and if it is to reach everyone in the population, it will do so when enough people emphasize the need for taking personal responsibility for health care: individuals by actively promoting health, and physicians and other health professionals by actively increasing their roles in solving local problems. An important first step would be to give back to physicians the power to make decisions regarding what is best for patient health. Government cost control strategists and others who interfere in the choices, directly or indirectly, have threatened the very quality of medicine.

Another problem which is plaguing the quality of health care is the age old problem of greed.

The best antidote to greed is to demonstrate the enduring value of charity and sharing. Volunteerism can make a big difference. If physicians were to offer some of their services to public aid clinics or to those unable to afford the total cost of their health care, the public would recognize the commitment. In an environment in which physicians took a leading role in supporting their communities, attitudes toward the medical profession would soon change and the public would again look upon medical doctors with a sense of appreciation and admiration.

One of the things we are doing at *Making Medicine Work* is to emphasize how volunteerism can solve some of the problems of medical care. Here are some comments about a few of our projects:

THE ALEXIAN PROJECT©

The Alexian Project was started at the Alexian Brothers Hospital where I work. It encourages health care professionals to donate private practice time to treat individuals and families who are unable to afford medical care and treatment. Health care professionals are invited to share in the joy of giving to their profession and their community by providing free health care to the needy. I contribute one full morning a month to seeing patients at the local hospital. Physicians with other specialities make similar contributions from their offices so that a broad spectrum of patients can receive free care. At one time, many of these patients would have been seen in my private practice and their expenses would have been covered by public aid. But I found that it was such a hassle to handle the forms and government red tape that I prefer to see them for free rather than waste my time and my staff's energy on handling the paper work.

Physicians and other health care professionals who would like information about giving voluntary time can contact *Making Medicine Work* to learn about how to set up similar projects.

THE STAR PROJECT©

While the indigent often need to receive health care through government services or in totally free clinics, young families with children are another example of a population at risk of not receiving adequate health care. Many Americans—steady wage earners among the working poor—find that they cannot afford to meet medical payments on a budget which barely gets them through the month. The Star Project provides a solution for these individuals and for physicians who are trying to avoid the headache of HMOs. Under the project, people earning roughly $30,000 a year or less, whether insured or uninsured, will be screened by the project's staff and placed on a sliding scale, receiving reductions in physician's fees of up to 90 percent, based upon ability to pay. Those without insurance will be given incentive to purchase low-cost policies which cover hospitalization and outpatient testing.

This project also offers health care professionals an alternative to participating in health maintenance organizations. Although HMOs reimburse at about the same rate as our sliding scale, paperwork is eliminated and fees are paid at the time of service. The greatest benefit is to the patients who would not otherwise receive quality medical care, but the project will also generate good will for both the doctors involved and the medical profession in general.

THE PATIENT AWARENESS PROGRAM©

How many times have patients left their doctor's offices feeling as though they have not had their questions adequately answered? How often do patients feel as though physicians have not considered their feelings or fears in prescribing a medication or a regimen? Conversely, how many times have doctors felt as if their patients wanted solutions without making any commitment to their own well-being? The *Patient*

146

Awareness Program addresses these issues by offering seminars about getting the most out of health care. A videotape seminar is available for individuals and groups.

THE MEDICAL SCHOOL PROJECT©

The Medical School Project addresses the problem that medical or other health care students face in making the transition from classroom to examination room. We are designing courses to help students understand the human side of medicine and to learn how to intelligently utilize and disseminate the scientific information which health care professionals must master. The program is designed to promote the concept that good health care depends upon a partnership between healer and patient.

It is important to understand that *Making Medicine Work* is not a club or an organization in the ordinary sense; it has no dues. While the organization does accept donations because expenses are incurred in promoting its programs, we would much rather have an individual work at the solution to a problem than merely send in a donation. The reason is simple: our philosophy is based on the assumption that the best contribution anyone can make is to directly work at solving a problem. If a person were merely to offer a donation and then not look around for ways to help solve local problems, that act would be an avoidance of the very responsibility we are trying to promote.

Let me now report on the efforts of other individuals who have made a contribution to improving medical care by employing creative solutions to problems. The following examples are but a few of the many wonderful programs and efforts which we have heard about since beginning *Making Medicine Work*. These samples are offered, partly to disseminate information and partly to stimulate the reader to be creative in seeking solutions to local problems.

Physician Bob Swartz

Bob Swartz is a highly successful plastic surgeon who, just a short time ago, was experiencing burnout. He admits that, though he did not hate his job, "it was not something that gave me a great deal of satisfaction." Then a friend encouraged Bob to make a trip to the Philippines for the purpose of helping people who were not receiving adequate medical care. Although he resisted for quite some time, Bob finally agreed to go. Ironically, heavy fighting in the Philippines forced the trip to be canceled, and Bob felt as if he had been given the excuse he was looking for to avoid the trip. His schedule, after all, was full. But when the call came again, he rearranged his schedule and went anyway—even though he admits that his motivation "didn't have anything to do with the virtue of helping people; it was as much a matter of not wanting to look bad in front of friends."

The trip, however, changed Bob's life—for the better. He performed operations to correct cleft palates and other physical abnormalities for young children. The effort gave Bob a totally new perspective on his own problems and stress. During operations in the Philippines, the electricity or the water were liable to go out in the middle of an operation, yet Bob learned how to get through the difficulties. The experience made him learn to accept and more readily cope with the slight inconveniences and problems of the modern operating room. So he developed greater patience and an appreciation for the advantages we have. More than anything, what he was doing gave him a new sense of commitment to his profession. Bob says, "I felt more pride in being a physician. I had lost the realization that being a plastic surgeon was something special. I am not trying to be arrogant, but I do have some special skills—and that is a good thing. A person should enjoy the fact that he has some knowledge or skill that can help other people."

For Bob Swartz, service has altered his life. He has been renewed and he is making a contribution—regularly—to young children who would never have the opportunity or the resources to receive care were it not for Bob's generosity. Since his first trip to the Philippines, Bob has been to Thailand and to Honduras, and he intends to keep making this service a part of his yearly work. His commitment is bringing hope to hundreds; one man is making a contribution to many and he is doing it for free. Of course, as he freely admits, he has been repaid in ways which transcend any monetary reward.

One of Bob's greatest regrets is that, though he would like to offer the same type of service in the United States, the present system simply makes it impossible—because of the threat of malpractice litigation.

Opticare

In Phoenix, Arizona, Opticare is an organization which works with physicians in the interest of helping the public at large receive good eye health care. Much of their work benefits the elderly. Opticare's story is important because it demonstrates that health care professionals with different specialities can work together in the interest of the public. The organization was started because a young eye doctor was moving into an area which was close to saturated with eye care professionals, and he needed to know what portion or segment of the population was not being served. What he discovered was that in an area heavily populated by senior citizens, fully half had not seen an eye professional in five years. Surveys told him that the senior citizens were, in fact, worried about their eyes and realized the need for care. But the elderly population was very, very skeptical of doctors and so they avoided making visits even though they had fears for their vision. One very serious concern for them was a fear of losing their drivers' licenses due to poor vision. But even though most drove, they tried to drive only short distances, which was itself a limiting factor in seeing eye care professionals. Setting up appointments and driving across town in heavy traffic to an appointment was frightening to most. They had other fears besides: one was that they did not understand deductibles, Medicare, insurance forms, the potential expenses, and the like. They were afraid of being ripped off, overcharged for whatever treatment they would receive. And, of course, they feared they would hear those horrible words that they were going blind; many spoke of the threat of blindness in the same way they might talk about cancer. The result was that a large segment of the population was not receiving the care necessary for preventing blindness, a truly tragic situation because the majority of eye problems which lead to blindness are fully treatable.

A creative solution was called for. Opticare 2000 was formed, and a number of vision specialists who would normally have competed with each other designed a benefits package which would reach those very citizens who, stymied by their fears, were not receiving protection. First of all, they offered free evaluations, not in their own clinics but in places where elderly citizens would normally congregate: churches, retirement centers, and the like. During these evaluations, the staff was sensitive not to frighten the individuals being screened. Those patients who had an actual or a potential problem were urged to make appointments with their doctors, whether or not the eye doctors were part of the sponsoring group. If the individuals being screened did not have a doctor, they were given the opportunity to make an appointment. Their needs were taken into consideration. Those who had difficulty with language barriers would be sent somewhere where they could be helped by a bilingual staff. Some would be offered free transportation because they had difficulty or fears concerning driving. And, of course, advice and counsel regarding insurance forms was always offered. Cheryl Holmes, who works with the group, indicates that the free screenings are not a factory production line affair. Only eight or ten seniors are seen at any one screening, and all are given a thorough checkup which takes roughly fifteen minutes. Everyone benefits from this arrangement. The senior citizens who have fears which prevent them from seeking help get evaluations for free. If they have no problems, they have spent nothing. If they will face a serious problem which could lead to blindness or increasingly poor vision, they receive counsel for free and can seek help at their own option, not necessarily with a member of the sponsoring group. The whole community wins. By going to the senior citizens and offering their service for free, Opticare 2000 has lessened the fears and helped save the vision of many elderly citizens.

Cheryl Holmes' most enthusiastic comments were reserved for a new project which was initiated by the group. Research done just a few years ago suggested that ultraviolet light is probably a contributing factor in producing cataracts. Some researchers feel that the issue is even more significant for seniors because the eyes of elderly people are not as resilient in repairing damage caused by ultraviolet light. So Opticare 2000 began providing elderly citizens with free ultraviolet goggles which fit over glasses. Cheryl was so proud of the program because it prevents problems rather than correcting them. She says: "Keep in mind that doctors, particularly ophthamologists, make their money, most of their money, by doing surgery, and yet our membership supported us totally on preventing the very problem which produces their income."

Center for Attitudinal Change

Physicians are not alone in making volunteer contributions to those in need of health care. In Chicago, I recently met Judith Butler who, with a group of non-physician volunteers, runs the non-profit Center For Attitudinal Change, a clinic and outreach center which helps those in need. The Center work is based on the writings of Gerald Jampolsky, who recommends using love and release from fear as methods of healing.

The Clinic offers counseling to rape victims, AIDS and HIV positive patients, and victims of child abuse. The counseling services the clinic provides are free of charge, and the staff is volunteer. The same policy holds for the parent location in Tiburon, California.

Indeed, all across America, non-physicians are participating in volunteer work in various clinics, hospitals, nursing homes, and outreach centers. We should recognize the opportunity

154

for each of us to become involved and acknowledge these unsung heroes of the world who
make such a difference in the quality of life for
so many.

Physician Howard Homler

Howard Homler is another physician who, in
spite of being an excellent clinical diagnostician,
felt incomplete in his work, frustrated that he
was "doing patchwork medicine." An internist,
he would, for example, send his patients to
surgery to have infected organs or cancerous
growths removed, only to see these same
patients revert to bad habits and not avoid the
conditions which produced their problems. In
his own words, Howard says, "Although I was
superb at making unusual diagnoses and manag-
ing real tough cases, I found that, for me, I was
missing a whole side of patient relations—that is,
really communicating with people and having
them feel well. I was being very parental, telling
patients what to do, what they shouldn't be
doing, but not really having an experience of
producing well-being for them—where they
could really do something for their own health
and feel good about it."
Howard began to analyze why so many
patients were not improving as well as they
might and he began to rethink the doctor-patient

155

relationship. He says, "We face a real problem in the medical profession. Most patients do not do what the doctor tells them to do. One person, the doctor, acts like an expert, and the other person, the patient, is treated as someone who just doesn't know and needs to be told what to do—just like a parent telling a child. The pattern is the result of receiving training in the medical and chemical aspects of health rather than on the background of a relationship between doctor and patient. Even our language betrays our attitude. When we talk of patients following instructions, we talk of compliance rates, rather than talking about cooperation."

Howard began to rethink his relationship to his patients when he realized that "the real reason why people come to doctors may have nothing to do with a specific ache or pain; the key to being a good physician is finding out what is really troubling the patient." So, in spite of being an excellent diagnostician, Howard realized that "our focus is on what is wrong, rather than what is right. We have the legal climate which makes us worry about not missing what we should have found, not making an error in diagnosis, but that is the wrong focus—the focus on disease, but not on wellness. In fact, the term wellness does not have much power in medicine nowadays. Usually, doctors assume it means the absence of disease; but, really, we know it means a lot more than that. Some of my cancer patients have more wellness than some of my patients who have nothing wrong with them.''

Howard has emphasized the maintenance of wellness. In fact, some of his most moving comments relate to what it means to be well. ''When I see patients with cancer suddenly realize how important their relationships with other people are and how great it is to be alive because they know they only have a certain amount of time to be alive—they have a special spark about being alive—well I call that wellness or vitality and it is just awe inspiring. And that is what I would love to impart to all patients: inspire those who are not terminally ill to recognize what they have. Someone with a sore throat should recognize that this will not last, that if he takes care of himself, he can soon feel well again. I know for me, I'm just delighted when patients are taking care of themselves. I just pat them on the back and say: if you need any suggestions or if anything is bothering you, just let me know, but it is great to see you doing so well on your own.''

One of the truly important breakthroughs in Howard's thinking was the breaking of old prejudices. When he was struggling with the question of why certain patients would not cease their bad habits, he began to wonder about other types of healers. Naturally skeptical of chiropractors, as many physicians are, he was amazed to find that their patients had great loyalty to them. "Chiropractors—I always thought they were just crazy, you know, yet these days we read in our medical literature just how often patients choose chiropractors for certain problems and get superb results." Sensitive to the monetary competition between health care practitioners, Howard decided to look into what chiropractors were offering. One of the first insights he gained was that chiropractors almost always promoted general health by emphasizing issues like good nutrition. They seemed to have far better success than medical doctors at being able to convince a patient to quit smoking or drinking because they brought a different attitude to their patients. Howard still has his questions and is still skeptical about some of the assertions and theories employed by chiropractors. As he says, "I don't think that it is necessarily appropriate for chiropractors to prescribe blood pressure medicines." Yet at the same time, he admits: "It's probably not appropriate for me to treat cases of low back pain with analgesics."

Rather than simply dismiss other health professionals, Howard began to organize get-togethers between health professionals from different disciplines: chiropractors, psychologists, nurses, surgeons, medical managers, and even legal experts. The purpose of the meetings was to learn about issues of health care and communication. Why, for example, in spite of the amazing technological advances, are patients often less satisfied with the system than in past centuries when the medical practices employed were, in light of modern knowledge, downright counter productive. Questions of patient superstitions and beliefs were raised, what their role was in healing or in causing patients to ignore their physicians' instructions. Doctors often send patients off, totally unaware of their unwillingness to accept a diagnosis, no matter how accurate it is. And Howard came to realize that physicians are superstitious too. Physicians, for example, are sometimes reluctant to treat AIDS patients out of fear, even though they know that AIDS is not easily transmittable; yet they will treat other patients with highly contagious diseases and not worry about the threat.

Howard Homler reflects the best ideals of someone in the health professions. Rather than close his mind to alternate approaches to promoting health, he has gone out of his way to learn from those he might ordinarily be skeptical of. In doing so, he has helped various professionals learn how they can benefit from alternate approaches and how they can promote responsibility in their patients. He has also gotten various professionals to think about their problems: what can one learn from the efforts that were not successful?

As I conclude this section on Howard Homler, I think it important to note that I am not advocating any forms of quackery. There is an awful lot of nonsense out there which passes for "medical" knowledge. Our most productive advances come from the application of the modern scientific method which has revealed the secrets of the human body. The understanding of the processes which keep us healthy helps us to deal with and treat disease. We must, as curious creatures, continue to research and build on our understanding. Physicians cannot be capable if they fail to master the science of their disciplines. But healing is also an art, and those who are best at it are those who have open minds, who are sensitive, and who can ask questions about what works in medicine and why.

I think the principles articulated in this book are applicable to more than medicine. In fact, they are an extension of the very best ideas upon which this nation was founded. The individual is assumed to be the best judge of his own well-being and is given maximum freedoms to choose his course of action in life, provided he does not violate the rights of others. This freedom carries with it the responsibility to be intelligent, to strive to know and understand in order to be able to make wise choices. We live in a democracy, in which our well-being and happiness are dependent on our personal efforts. If doctors assume all responsibility for their patients' well-being, or if patients depend totally on their doctors to correct their ills, then the system will not work.

Everywhere one looks, our culture seems to be losing precisely what the founding fathers said was necessary to make a nation thrive: individual responsibility. We turn to other people for our entertainment and our gratification; when we ask that a doctor give us health, we are asking the wrong guy. He can give advice and he can help minimize the impact of temporary disruptions like disease, but everyone must want to be well if they are to be well.

As I conclude this book then, I offer a challenge to all of its readers. I am not concerned ultimately whether or not you agree with everything I have said. But I would ask that you not put the book down without considering what you can do to help solve at least one corner of the nation's health crisis puzzle. Your solutions need not be mine. If you are a health care professional, ask yourself what will promote the well-being of your patients? Perhaps even ask questions like: what will make your job easier? Would the malpractice crisis in your community be eased if you, as an individual, were to invite doctors and lawyers to meet to discuss the situation? You may be surprised to find that such a meeting could promote understanding and serve as a source of recommendations to alleviate the crisis. If you are not a health professional, what do you intend to do to promote your own health? Is there any way you can help others, individuals or organizations, as they try to help fellow members in the community? The gesture may be simple—giving a pint of blood for the first time—but if you do something, you will be helping to "make medicine work," and you are to be thanked for your effort.

Frankly, although I may have offended some physicians in saying what I did in this book, I have one final defense of my assertions. The way I am practicing medicine now has put the fun back into my profession. When I was threatened and afraid of losing patients, when the increasing malpractice premiums made me feel insecure, I lost sight of what I had entered the profession for. Getting up and going to work was a chore; patients seemed to be threats; life was a drag. How many of my colleagues felt the same way? How we did grumble to each other! No more. Now I seek out physicians like myself who have altered their practices; we share a common feeling: we are happy and eager to be working with patients. When doctor and patient work in a partnership, when they are sensitive to each other and willing to listen, when they mutually discover how interesting human nature and the human body is, then life becomes a challenge and every healed patient a joyful blessing. That old bugaboo of so many white collar professions—burnout—has been replaced by an eagerness to greet every new day.

As I write these last words, I am vividly aware of my own mortality. Someday, I will serve patients no more. Yet that does not bother me; while I am here, I intend to do all I can to promote health and well-being. Being well is the essence and secret of leading a good life. It is, in fact, an essential part of morality. Health is one of the few things in life worth pursuing as an end in itself, for without it, it is difficult to promote other values. May you, the reader, have the good fortune to live in health and the good sense to preserve it.

YOUR PERSONAL INVITATION

You are invited to become part of MAKING MEDICINE WORK, the non-profit foundation dedicated to transforming health care in the world.

Our mailing address is 850 Biesterfield Road, Suite 3002, Elk Grove Village, Illinois, 60007. We can be reached at 1-800-848-4977.

Although we do need and appreciate financial support, we have no dues or memberships available. We invite you to contact us to see how you can create your own projects or foundation, either as a patient, physician, or health care worker. MAKING MEDICINE WORK can be a support system for you to create positive changes in the health care system. It is our belief that personal responsibility is more than just sending money to support an organization, but requires your personal commitment and action. In other words, you don't have to join the club, you just have to do it!

We will also be glad to send you information regarding seminars available on videotape and additionally, information about the newsletter we are currently developing which will provide subscribers with timely information about MAKING MEDICINE WORK and the future of health care in both America and the world.

WORKING TOGETHER, WE CAN MAKE MEDICINE WORK!

Other books available by Breakthru Publishing—
"The Publisher Of Ideas Whose Time Has
Come:"

Diets Don't Work!

A breakthrough in losing weight when diets
fail.

The One Hour Orgasm

Everything your parents didn't know or teach
you about sex and relationships.

Diets Still Don't Work!

How to lose weight, step-by-step, even after
you've failed at dieting.

Copies are available through your local
bookstores or may be ordered directly by calling
1-800-227-1152.